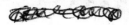

VIKING CANADA

BREAKING THE AGE BARRIER

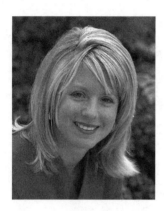

Sherry Torkos, BSc, Phm, is a nationally recognized pharmacist, author, and lecturer. She has written several health booklets, as well as articles for numerous publications, and is the author of *The Complete Idiot's Guide® to Women's Health for Canadians*. Sherry is a certified fitness instructor and health enthusiast who enjoys sharing her passions with others. As a health expert, Sherry is interviewed frequently on radio and appears regularly on CTV, CHTV, Global TV, and CityTV. She lives and practices holistic pharmacy in the Niagara region of Ontario. For more information, visit her at www.sherrytorkos.com.

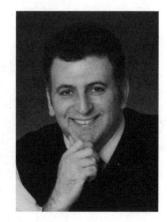

Farid Wassef, RPh, CCN, is a highly regarded pharmacist and certified clinical nutritionist who has published numerous articles in health magazines and medical journals. He serves as an advisory council member at the Institute for Functional Medicine and as an editorial board member for both the *Journal of the American Nutraceutical Association* and the *International Journal of Integrative Medicine*. He regularly counsels patients and conducts seminars for healthcare professionals and the public on healthy lifestyles, diet, nutrition, and natural medicine. He practices at Houston Pharmacy in Stouffville, Ontario. For more information, please visit prescription4nutrition.com.

Strategies for
Optimum Health,
Energy, and Longevity

BREAKING
THE AGE BARRIER

Sherry Torkos, BSc, Phm

Farid Wassef, RPh, CCN

VIKING
CANADA

VIKING CANADA

Published by the Penguin Group

Penguin Books, a division of Pearson Canada, 10 Alcorn Avenue, Toronto, Ontario, Canada M4V 3B2

Penguin Books Ltd, 80 Strand, London WC2R 0RL, England

Penguin Putnam Inc., 375 Hudson Street, New York, New York 10014, U.S.A.

Penguin Books Australia Ltd, 250 Camberwell Road, Camberwell, Victoria 3124, Australia

Penguin Books India (P) Ltd, 11, Community Centre, Panchsheel Park, New Delhi – 110 017, India

Penguin Books (NZ) Ltd, cnr Rosedale and Airborne Roads, Albany, Auckland 1310, New Zealand

Penguin Books (South Africa) (Pty) Ltd, 24 Sturdee Avenue, Rosebank 2196, South Africa

Penguin Books Ltd, Registered Offices: 80 Strand, London WC2R 0RL, England

First published 2003

10 9 8 7 6 5 4 3 2

This publication contains the opinions and ideas of its author and is designed to provide useful advice in regard to the subject matter covered. The herbs and other treatments in this book are described for the information and education of readers. They are not a replacement for diagnosis and treatment by qualified health professionals. The author and publisher are not engaged in rendering health or other professional services in this publication. This publication is not intended to provide a basis for action in particular circumstances without consideration by a competent professional. The author and publisher expressly disclaim any responsibility for any liability, loss, or risk, personal or otherwise, which is incurred as a consequence, directly or indirectly, of the use and application of any of the contents of this book.

Printed and bound in Canada on acid free paper.

National Library of Canada Cataloguing in Publication Data

Torkos, Sherry
        Breaking the age barrier / Sherry Torkos, Farid Wassef.

Includes bibliographical references and index.

ISBN 0-670-04346-X

1. Aging—Prevention. 2. Middle aged persons—Health and hygiene. I. Wassef, Farid, 1964- II. Title.

RA776.75.T67 2003   613'.0434   C2002-905009-X

Author photos:
Sherry Torkos: Copyright © Michael Dismatsek, Dismatsek Photographic
Farid Wassef: Copyright © Katherine Aczel

Visit Penguin Books' website at www.penguin.ca

BREAKING
THE AGE BARRIER

CONTENTS

ACKNOWLEDGEMENTS

I would like to thank pharmacists Mary and Abraam Rofael, Joyce Lummiss, Alma Timbers, and my staff for providing coverage at our pharmacy.

A special thanks to Jeff Bland for providing the Foreword. He is a tremendous human being and has been a great mentor to me. It is his tireless research efforts over the last 30 years that have allowed me to practice a type of medicine that has made a significant difference in the lives of my patients.

To my parents, Lou and Antoinette, for their enduring love and support that have kept me going throughout this entire project. A special thanks to them because they are most responsible for my growth and development as a person.

To my brothers, George and Edward, who have provided friendship and a sounding board for my often endless and ambitious ideas about health care.

In loving memory of my grandmother, Regina Mansour, who taught me about acceptance, love, and patience, and that they are all available with a faith in God. It is her wisdom that has given me the courage to pursue new possibilities in my profession. She remains a great source of inspiration.

To my loving wife, Peggy, who is most dear to me. She is directly responsible for the successful completion of this book. The road is often lonely when trying to bring forth new ideas. She has not only made it bearable but has also believed in my vision of better health care and that together we can make difference in our corner of the world. I could not have found a better friend on this journey.

Farid Wassef

I would like to gratefully acknowledge those individuals who helped and encouraged me during the writing of this book:

To Bill Steinburg, with sincere appreciation for all your help in researching and editing my manuscript. I appreciate the countless hours that you put into this project and your advice and encouragement throughout the writing process.

To Tanya Rouble, BSc, personal trainer, and close friend, I thank you for your contribution to the research and preparation of my exercise chapter. You have made such a difference in so many lives with your enthusiasm and passion for fitness and health.

To Dr. Joy Wright, BSc Phm, Pharm D, my friend and colleague, for your help in researching the content for the chapter on the immune system. I appreciate your help and support.

To my co-author, Farid, I would also like to extend my sincere thanks for your support, guidance, and encouragement throughout this process. You have inspired me in my own personal and professional development, and I am so pleased to have worked with you on this project.

To my partner, Rick, I thank you for your love, patience, and understanding while I have spent many long hours at my computer. Your ongoing help and support made this book possible.

To my parents, Karen and Joe, and all my family and friends, I thank you for always being there for me with support and encouragement. I am very fortunate to have a loving network of people in my life.

Farid and I would also like to extend our thanks to Judith Turnbull for her help in the final editing and to all the folks at Penguin Books for this opportunity.

Sherry Torkos

FOREWORD

In the past one hundred years, there have been three assumptions about disease that have characterized the development of Western medical practice. These assumptions are:

1. Aging produces chronic disease.

2. Disease is a result of infection, trauma, or flawed genes.

3. There is little a person can do to change the course of certain diseases if they have the genes for heart disease, cancer, diabetes, or arthritis.

Within the past decade, however, these three basic assumptions have all been proven incorrect. Aging has been shown not to cause any specific diseases. Chronic diseases are not just a result of flawed genes, trauma, or infection, but also a result of an inappropriate connection between genetic uniqueness and environmental factors. These environmental factors include diet, activity patterns, stress, and lifestyle choices.

The deciphering over the past decade of the "code of life" that is locked into our chromosomes has uncovered an unexpected observation. Our genes do not tell us how we are going to die, but rather how we should live to maximize our genetic potential and to get the optimal functional health from our genetic legacy.

This discovery will produce what Thomas Kuhn termed a "paradigm shift"—a major change in how the average person views the world. This revolution's impact on medicine will be like no other since Pasteur identified the origin of common communicable diseases as arising from infectious microbes, too small to be seen without the aid of a microscope.

In their excellent book *Breaking the Age Barrier,* Farid Wassef and Sherry Torkos convey how the average person can access the results of this paradigm shift in health and disease for their own lives. This book chronicles the nature of the health revolution that we are now undergoing, and explains how readers can leverage this information in constructing their own personalized health plans to maximize their genetic potential.

Health books are often built upon the experience of the authors and not properly grounded in a firm understanding of the latest breakthroughs in biological sciences. That is not the case with this book. As pharmacists who have specialized in functional medicine, Farid Wassef and Sherry Torkos know what is happening at the forefront of nutritional and biomedical sciences. As pharmacists, too often they have seen the results of over-dependence on the power of the prescription pad to deliver good health. The over-use of medications has resulted in its own disorders, termed "Iatrogenic diseases" or those conditions caused by adverse side-effects of long-term medication.

Wassef and Torkos have written a book that can and should be used to help the reader take advantage of these exciting 21st century medical developments. This book gives us the information we need on how we should treat our genes to enjoy good health and a sustained level of function throughout the whole of our lives. I believe that anyone applying the principles described in *Breaking the Age Barrier* will be rewarded with improved functional health at any age.

Jeffrey S. Bland, PhD, FACN, CNS,
author of the bestselling book, Genetic Nutritioneering

INTRODUCTION

"Aging is inevitable." Even though just about everybody would agree with this statement, the average life expectancy of human beings has become a subject of intense inquiry. As health educators, we have combed through the wealth of data that has emerged in the medical sciences. From this, we have selected the most reliable new theories and facts that explain how and why people age. In the chapters that follow, we will present this new information to you.

Asking the Right Questions

Most of us feel that we each have a predetermined health path. But do we really need to repeat the patterns that ruled our parents? Are we bound by our genetic inheritance? Can we edit our genes and rewrite the future chapters of our lives? Better yet, can we maintain the vigor and vitality of our youth across our life span? Can good health be an enduring feature of a fulfilled and contented life? Are age-related diseases a necessary by-product of growing old? This book will explore and answer these and many other questions.

In North America, age-related diseases and chronic maladies have generally been treated with prescription medicines. In these pages, however, we will look at a more integrative and comprehensive approach. On the basis of extensive research and clinical experience, we have come to believe that health problems associated with aging are treatable and often avoidable. If you follow the guidelines in this book, your health should improve, no matter what your current physical state or age. Be ready to take action.

Waiting for Tomorrow

Many people believe that with the unraveling of the human genome modern medicine will soon be able to correct genetic errors. The mere insertion of "good genes," it is thought, will help people triumph over the inconveniences of aging. There is also a kind of blind faith that one day soon a collection of new medicines will shield us from the salvos of aging. While these expectations may or may not be realistic, we can safely say that we are still several generations away from their becoming a reality.

Many have also taken hope from the recent discovery that the human body has enough restorative genetic material to put the maximum human life span in the range of 120–140 years and possibly beyond. Still, no one has yet outlined how such longevity can be achieved. Don't get caught waiting on the sidelines for the hypothetical to become a reality.

Natural Aging

No one can escape his or her mortality. And given what is currently understood about genetic inheritance, an individual's maximum life span may be fixed. But what if the amount of time people spend in faltering health could be compressed into the last few days of their lives rather than stretched across decades? Many researchers contend that, irrespective of genetics, we can increase our "health span" by maximizing the number of years we are fully functional and in a state of good health.[1]

We tend to suffer more diseases as we age because of a loss of organ reserves. When we are 22, we can readily mobilize our reserves to overcome threats to our health. Once most of us reach 72, however, our chances of rebounding quickly from pneumonia, say, or a bone fracture are sadly diminished, as we have fewer reserves to draw upon. Thus, to ensure healthy aging, it is extremely important to prevent the loss of organ reserves.

Chronic and debilitating diseases not only drain our organ reserves but also accelerate our rate of aging. We all know someone who is chronologically 45 but has the joints of an 80-year-old. Conversely, some 65-year-olds have the zest and zeal to run six miles. Why is this so?

Chronic inflammation and free-radical damage is the thread that connects all age-related diseases, with the most salient features being pain and fatigue. These warning signs are dismissed as part of the normal aging processes—but they are not normal. Why, then, do millions of people cut back on their regular activities as they age? It is our belief that they do so unnecessarily, that advancing years need not bring us disease and significant loss of function. In this book, we will discuss how you can prevent the avoidable and delay the inevitable during the aging process.

A Matter of Genes

Our contentions are based on scientific data as well as on what we learned while examining individuals who had successfully made it to a healthy 100 years or more. These individuals helped us discover a host of common factors behind healthy aging. They did not owe their longevity to some secret trick or to a particular collection of genes. In fact, no single gene has been identified to explain who will remain intact as they grow old. And that's good news, since it suggests that healthy aging is available to almost everyone.

In the chapters ahead, we will look at what it means to age naturally and remain healthy. We will also define what we mean by good health. Good health, of course, is more than the absence of disease; it is a sense of physical, mental, and social well-being, a state of mind and body that allows an individual to cope successfully with challenges to health and remain functional. Healthy aging allows an individual to develop a sense of purpose, and this ultimately results in fulfillment.

Creating Inspiration

Yes, aging is inevitable, but disease is not. Imagine being able to respond more effectively to the stresses of life. Imagine having the energy to pursue what your heart desires. We ask you to leave behind your anxiety about growing old and embrace a better possibility.

As health educators, we have been inspired by the fact that all diseases and the aging process itself share a significant number of features. Furthermore, despite our genetic diversity, most of what influences the expression of our genes is modifiable. All this translates into new expectations about aging.

This book is meant to be explored, but it also invites participation. The chapters are purposely arranged, building upon a foundation. Read them in order, for in doing so you will be able to adapt the information to your own situation. For example, you will be able to design for yourself an ideal diet, lifestyle, and nutritional supplement regime. Write your own prescription for achieving a functional state of health for the full length of your life.

Remember, your current health status is the result of everything that has washed over your genes thus far. How you are today is only one of the several outcomes that were once available to you. There is an incredible potential in your gene pool. Read further to learn about the many factors you can incorporate into your life to shape a new you. With a well-nourished physical body and spirit, you will be able to deal readily with aging and not be battered by it. This book, based as it is on scientific evidence, will help you conclude that it is possible to "break the age barrier."

PART 1

FACTS ABOUT AGING

1

PERSPECTIVES ON HEALTH AND AGING

Take a few seconds and imagine what it might be like to wake up some day 40 years from now. What would you awaken to? What would your health be like? Let's say you spring up out of bed with incredible verve on this future day. You feel vitally alive, ready to work, and confident that you still have a lot to offer. The sunrise inspires you. You marvel at the splendor of nature and feel invigorated after your morning stroll. Unencumbered with poor health, you feel free to pursue the activities that mean so much to you. On this day you feel there is still a lot to be explored and experienced. On this day you feel alive.

Most of you will now be saying, "Wait a minute. I don't even feel that way now." That may be true, but can the kind of health you do have endure the passage of time? Physical, mental, emotional, and spiritual wellness determines your state of health, and life can erect many barriers between you and healthy aging. An examination of current health statistics will help us identify specific barriers.

Probabilities

In the United States the average life expectancy for men is 73.6 years; for women it is 79.4 years.[1] In Canada men can expect to live 75.7 years and women 81.4 years.[2] The majority of men and women in North America will be around in their eighth decade. Moreover, a significant percentage of the population will live to the age of 90 and beyond. The 21st century promises every succeeding generation a longer average life span than that of the previous one.

Contributing to such longevity are better hygienic practices, survival from childhood illness, and modern medicine's victories over the life-threatening infectious diseases that plagued society 100 years ago. In addition, the grave nutritional diseases that prevented proper growth and development are now a rarity.

So, can all of this be perceived as good news? Well, it's good but it's not the whole picture. While increased life expectancy indicates an overall improvement in the health of a population, it does not reveal the *quality* of health that individuals enjoy during their life span.

Barriers to Good Health

As we age, the most significant barrier to having sterling health is heart and circulatory disease. Collectively named cardiovascular disease, this age-related health barrier often results in heart attack and stroke; it is the number one cause of death, disability, and illness, affecting nearly 50 percent of the population.[3] Cardiovascular disease affects men and women equally, and its onset can be in individuals as young as 15.

Cancer is the second leading cause of death in North America.[4] Prostate cancer is the most commonly diagnosed cancer in men, breast cancer in women. Collectively, millions of potential years of life are lost due to this disease in any single year.

Closing in on the two biggest barriers to good health is adult-onset or Type 2 diabetes. In Type 2 diabetes, poorly functioning insulin metabolism makes it hard for the body to control blood-sugar levels. In Type 1 diabetes, the pancreas is unable to produce insulin, making daily injections of this hormone a necessity. Both types of diabetes are major causes of heart disease and the most common reasons for limb amputation, kidney failure, and blindness. Fifteen years from now, the number of diabetics will easily triple. The surging, age-related Type 2 diabetes is responsible for this projection, obesity being a leading risk factor.[5]

Accumulation of body fat and loss of muscle mass with each passing decade are other age-related problems. In North America over a third of the population are considered to be obese and another third overweight. Those not at their ideal body weight have greatly increased risks of developing heart disease, cancer, and diabetes.[6]

Loss of Function

One consistent finding among adults is that the incidence of loss of functional health increases with age. The most common physical disabilities are hearing and vision loss and muscle and joint problems. Those suffering from such disabilities may be unable to walk unassisted or perform the daily activities of independent living; the assistance of family members may be required. When significant cognitive (or mental) deficiency sets in as well, some direct form of medical intervention is necessary. Many such sufferers may spend their remaining years in a nursing home.

Consequences of Chronic Inflammation

Today only about 25 percent of the population 12 years of age and older rate their physical and mental health as excellent. Sadly, when people under 40 are excluded, this percentage shrinks. A host of chronic diseases is responsible for these abysmal statistics. Back problems and arthritis restrict the activities of millions; asthma, allergies, chronic fatigue syndrome, fibromyalgia, irritable bowel syndrome, and migraines are other examples of the increasingly common ailments that place limitations on a person's health.

All chronic diseases have the biological side effect of accelerating the rate of aging, and most such conditions are the result of uncontrolled inflammation and subsequent free-radical damage. By destroying cells, tissues, and organs, chronic inflammation leads to rapid aging. Pain and fatigue are the most significant symptoms of the chronic inflammatory process, which includes aging itself. Chronic inflammation is the reason many of us become increasingly achy and tired as we age.

People today tend to rely on prescription drugs to manage age-related diseases and chronic maladies. An astounding two-thirds of the population take medication to control pain, making pain management the main reason for medication use. Think of the number of pills your parents have taken daily as they've aged—this represents your genetic potential to have the same fate.

Breaking Genetic Molds

Genes are capable of carrying a multitude of messages. Inheriting a collection of genes responsible for heart disease does not mean you'll necessarily get it. Though you may be at a greater than average risk, other genes in your genetic book are also waiting to be read. Your life has many possible stories, not just one. Together, all these stories make up your genetic potential.

You are not at the mercy of your genes, for to a great extent you can control which genes are read and what they will say. This means that genetic expression is modifiable. Most importantly, healthy old age and its opposite, diseased aging, are not solely the products of genetic fate. Genetic expression is largely shaped by how you deal with stress, what you eat, your mental attitudes, and your emotional state—to mention just a few factors. Despite your genes, you can have good health.

A Compass for Good Health

Subsequent chapters contain a wealth of information about how to obtain a kind of health you probably never thought possible. You will be given strategies for coping with stress, for example. You'll learn how different lifestyles accelerate the aging process. You'll come to understand how your own lifestyle and habits may predispose you to age-related diseases that can become chronic. You will learn about the tremendous influence that food has on your health. You will be given sound nutritional advice. You will discover what parts of your body are especially vulnerable to the consequences of aging and how to give your body the support it needs. If your body has the right support, your physical, mental, and spiritual health will improve.

Natural aging is not synonymous with disease. In the pages ahead, we will look at the mechanisms that influence the rate of aging. These are the same mechanisms that bring about chronic disease. You will learn how your biochemistry can be manipulated to ensure healthy aging. Such manipulation can arrest and sometimes reverse chronic diseases. Rather than face ill health in the last 30 to 40 years of your life, you can look forward to a longer health span—that is, to good health in these final decades.

Conclusion

We started out by getting you to imagine your own good health 40 years from now. What you do today with your life can create that future. There are two things that we cannot give you to help you do this: resolve and time. You are the one who must first resolve to have better health, and you are the one who must make the time to pursue this course. This book will then enable you to design a program that will lead to the best possible health story for you.

2

WHY AND HOW WE AGE

This chapter will explore what causes the changes typically seen during the aging process. You will learn that no single mechanism is responsible for why and how people age. Many factors, in fact, contribute to healthy and diseased aging. It is important that you be aware of all of them. The purpose of this chapter, then, is to help you develop a well-rounded approach to enduring health.

Why Do We Age?

From the moment of birth, aging allows us to grow and develop physically. Aging also gives us the opportunity to mature mentally, emotionally, and spiritually. Since most of us have the innate capacity to learn from experience, getting older can mean getting wiser. Many of us, however, see the aging process not as an opportunity but as a burden, as something regrettable. We celebrate youth and fear growing old. We see aging as a degenerative process, marked by disease and disability. We fear that at some point society will have no use for us and we will be brushed aside.

Perhaps our greatest fear is that we will have no control over the changes that will occur in our bodies over time. Let's take a tour of the factors within our control that influence the rate at which we age.

Variables That Affect the Rate of Aging

Would your friends believe you if you claimed to be 20 years younger than you are? When we notice that people look younger or older than their actual age, we are observing the rate at which they are biologically aging. The most obvious signs associated with aging are wrinkles, graying and thinning hair, a decrease in muscle mass and tone, weight gain, and loss of teeth. Why do some people look more worn out than others as they get older?

The Wear and Tear Theory

In 1882 August Weismann, a German biologist, introduced the Wear and Tear Theory to explain the changes seen in aging and the variability in the rate at which people age. Our cells, tissues, and organs are damaged through overuse and abuse of the body. Not getting enough sleep, rest, or relaxation, consuming too much fat and sugar, and developing a dependence on caffeine, alcohol, nicotine, or other drugs are just some of the ways we abuse our bodies.

Exposure to environmental toxins can also damage us. The U.S. Environmental Protection Agency has estimated that over 100,000 man-made chemicals circulate among us, with several hundred added each year.[1] All these chemicals, either individually or in combination, are poisonous to the body at certain levels. With this kind of exposure, the body wears itself out in its attempt to detoxify itself.

Scores of other environmental stresses threaten our health. Emerging resistant strains of bacteria, viruses, parasites, and fungi are beginning to handcuff our immune system, causing chronic or recurring infections. The inappropriate use and overuse of antibiotics in medicine and agriculture have been largely blamed for this.

In addition, chronic mental and emotional stress can lead to problems like depression, ulcers, headaches, high blood pressure, and insomnia, all of which wear down the body. We are designed to handle many different types of stress, but not on a continuous basis. When we are young, our ability to respond and adapt to stress, deal with emotional trauma, sustain physical injury, and recover from infection is at its optimum. The essence of the Wear and Tear Theory is that our capacity to heal—our "healing force"—diminishes as we age. Eventually, poor lifestyle habits, the burden of toxins, microbial infections, and persistent stress wear down the body beyond repair. Weismann said it best: "Death occurs because a worn out tissue cannot forever renew itself."[2]

The Rate of Living Theory

In 1908, after studying the relationship between metabolic rate, body size, and longevity, German physiologist Max Rubner proposed the Rate of Living Theory of Aging. According to this theory, we are each born with a limited amount of energy. Our rate of aging, then, is determined by how quickly or slowly we use our allotted supply. The expression "Live fast and die young" sums up this theory. Spending all our energy in our youth leaves us with an "empty gas tank" as an adult; aging becomes an accelerated trip and quite possibly one fraught with disease. No doubt there is some truth to this; we can all think of times in our lives when we expended too much energy and in the process aged ourselves.

Both of the above theories are true, but neither explains why some people in your office fall victim to the flu that's going around while others stay healthy. And why do some people breeze through stressful situations, others develop ulcers or get headaches, and, worse yet, some develop heart disease? Moreover, why do some people maintain adequate energy levels as they age while others become increasingly fatigued?

The Free-Radical Theory

Modern-day theories have focused on biochemical processes inside our cells to explain individual differences in the rate of aging. Dr. Denham Harman, a physician and researcher at the University of Nebraska Medical Center, introduced the Free-Radical Theory of Aging in the 1950s.

Free radicals are unstable molecules, and left unchecked, they are capable of altering metabolism and damaging our bodies. They are a natural by-product of the body's normal metabolism. Certain environmental substances also act directly or indirectly as free radicals. Heavy metals, chemical solvents, pesticides, infectious microbes, drugs, alcohol, and cigarette smoke are some examples. Just as important, constant psychological and emotional stress can liberate free radicals to wreak havoc upon us.

Free radicals damage the body by exposing it to oxidative stress (a damaging chemical reaction). The inability to deal with oxidative stress has been blamed for aging and many age-related problems, among them Alzheimer's, arthritis, cancer, cardiovascular disease, cataracts, diabetes, and macular degeneration (an eye disease that leads to loss of eyesight). It is now recognized that aging and all chronic degenerative diseases involve both a surplus of free radicals and chronic inflammation. The two are inextricably linked: free radicals can initiate chronic inflammation, and chronic inflammation can produce free radicals. A vicious circle indeed.

Fortunately, the body has an antioxidant defense system. *Glutathione* is the major molecule found inside our cells that disarms free radicals before they cause problems. In the elderly, high levels of glutathione are associated with lower body weight, lower cholesterol, lower blood pressure, fewer illnesses, and higher levels of self-rated health. Seniors with the lowest levels of glutathione suffer from heart disease, arthritis, diabetes, or combinations thereof. [3]

Improving your body's ability to handle the load of free radicals raises your chances of aging healthily and avoiding disease. There are a number of ways to do this. One of the best is to increase the amount of vitamins, minerals, and other nutrients in your diet. Well over 4,000 phytochemicals (plant-based chemicals) have been identified in fruits, vegetables, and whole grains; these not only protect you against free-radical damage but also improve immune function, balance hormones, control inflammation, prevent cancer, and promote overall health.[4] (See Appendix 2.1.) Other evidence shows that antioxidant supplements and compounds derived from natural plants can be used to treat and even prevent a variety of age-related diseases.[5]

The Loss of Energy Theory

The Free-Radical Theory of Aging has become a central biochemical explanation for both aging and chronic degenerative disease. This has led researchers to explore the microscopic filaments in the cell known as *mitochondria*; it is in the mitochondria that free-radical production is the greatest and most significant. Every human cell contains anywhere from several hundred to a few thousand mitochondria. Just as heat is produced in the furnace in your home, energy is created in the mitochondria. The protein, carbohydrates, and fats derived from the foods you eat are shuttled into mitochondria and burned in the presence of oxygen to create energy.

The mitochondria need to produce enough energy to sustain the function of the body's key organs, glands, and systems. The heart, brain, liver, kidneys, adrenals, pancreas, and immune system have especially high energy requirements. Furthermore, a consistent supply of energy is needed for reparative processes and to detoxify and pump waste out of the cells of the body. It is thus easy to see why researchers take a great interest in mitochondria. Cardiovascular diseases, cancer, diabetes, Parkinson's, Alzheimer's, and even chronic fatigue syndrome and fibromyalgia are examples of the over 100 diseases directly linked to defects in mitochondrial function.[6] If enough mitochondria inside a cell decay and eventually die, the cell's energy requirements cannot be met and its death ensues. If enough of the cells that make up tissue die, then organs, glands, and various systems stop functioning. Increased fatigue and loss of function during the aging process are the initial warning signs that your mitochondria are failing.

Various nutrients preserve and even improve mitochondrial function—supplemental B vitamins, alpha lipoic acid, coenzyme Q10, acetyl-L-carnitine, L-carnitine, N-acetyl-cysteine, magnesium, and nicotinamide adenine dinucleotide (NADH).[7] But before putting supplements like these on your grocery list, read on so that you'll understand the whole story.

The Hormonal Decline Theory

The idea that the decline of hormones is a cause of aging was set in motion during the 1920s. The theory was that the fires of our youth are linked to high levels of various hormones in our bodies. Therefore, taking supplemental hormones as our natural supply gradually declines will restore the hormone levels of youth, slow down aging, and prevent disease.

Today, hormone replacement therapy (HRT) is the dominant medical strategy based on this theory. However, aside from treating the symptoms of aging, HRT has fallen short of its promise. Increased risks of blood clots, heart disease, stroke, and cancer are now associated with HRT.

The decline of hormones is a symptom—not a cause—of aging. Therefore, hormone supplements alone won't keep you unscathed during the aging process. That would be just too easy. What we need to do is get to the cause(s) of the decline in hormones and understand how hormones interact with one another.

The Neuroendocrine Theory

Vladimir Dilman, a Russian gerontologist, investigated the dynamic hormonal interplay that occurs in the body as it ages. In the 1950s he proposed the Neuroendocrine Theory to explain what causes accelerated aging and age-related diseases. Specifically, he studied how the nervous system works with the endocrine glands (these glands secrete into the bloodstream or lymph system the hormones that regulate all physiological processes).

To understand how the nervous system functions with the endocrine system, consider how your thermostat controls the temperature in your home, keeping it within a comfortable range. With time and overuse, the thermostat loses the ability to regulate the temperature properly. It has trouble sensing the actual temperature and turning the furnace on or off appropriately. The action of a thermostat captures the essence of the Neuroendocrine Theory. The hypothalamus gland, located in the brain, can be thought of as a thermostat; it controls body temperature, hunger, and thirst (among many other things) as well as how we respond to stress. Stress in all forms—mental, emotional, physical—has an impact on the hypothalamus. When the hypothalamus is stimulated, it activates the pituitary (this gland secretes hormones that control growth, reproduction, and various other of the body's activities), which in turn activates the adrenal glands (these glands secrete adrenaline and cortisol). The hypothalamus, pituitary, and adrenal glands are known as the *HPA axis*.

The Adrenal Glands

The HPA axis is the system used by the body to respond and adapt to stress. Cortisol is the major hormone produced and secreted by the adrenal glands that allows us to deal with situations that excite or frighten us. Imagine being in a state of continuous excitement or fear. Your HPA axis would be sent into overdrive, producing more and more cortisol as well as adrenaline. Too much cortisol can lead to hypertension, obesity, and elevated levels of cholesterol and blood sugar; it can also weaken the immune system and cause depression and memory loss.

The Hypothalamus

A healthy hypothalamus—considered to be the master gland of the endocrine system—can sense elevated levels of cortisol and responds by shutting off its production. However, with age and overexposure to various stressors, the hypothalamus loses this ability. To compensate, the adrenal glands crank out more cortisol in an attempt to get the hypothalamus to respond by shutting down the HPA axis, thereby preserving its function. Each and every time the hypothalamus is flooded with cortisol, it loses some of its ability to listen to the shut-down message. The ensuing vicious circle exhausts the adrenal glands. Over time they shrivel and die. When the adrenal glands lose significant function, you become excessively vulnerable to stress and experience chronic fatigue as well as pain from uncontrollable inflammation.

The root problem is the hypothalamus's loss of sensitivity to cortisol. In accelerated and diseased aging, cortisol levels rise steadily. In fact, apart from insulin, cortisol is the only hormone that rises during aging. The continuous engagement of the HPA axis and poor cortisol regulation are thus at the heart of Dilman's Neuroendocrine Theory of Aging. As a result of the overtaxing of the HPA axis, the other three regulatory systems ("axes") in the jurisdiction of the hypothalamus can begin to fail—specifically, the reproductive (hypothalamic-pituitary-gonadal), metabolic (hypothalamic-pituitary-thyroid), and immune (pineal-hypothalamic-pituitary-thymus) systems. When the end gland in each axis (gonads, thyroid, and thymus) loses significant function, the respective systems that are regulated fail.

The Gonads With age, the gonads, which include the testicles and ovaries, sputter in their ability to maintain ideal levels of testosterone and estrogen respectively. As a result, fertility is reduced and there is an increased likelihood of brain aging, muscle and bone loss, fat accumulation, and heart disease for both men and women. Interestingly, if the size and function of the adrenal glands can be maintained, they can compensate by producing these male and female hormones at the time of menopause and andropause (the time in a man's life when he experiences a decline in overall mental and physical health that can affect libido and stamina). However, when the HPA axis is continually operating on high and adrenal function cannot be maintained, this does not occur.

The Thyroid When the function of the thyroid gland becomes sub par, overall metabolism is affected. Digestion is sluggish and the body's ability to burn food completely for energy is impaired. The thyroid gland also plays a part in controlling body temperature, and one of the most obvious signs of an underactive thyroid is feeling cold. Hypothyroidism has been deemed a silent illness of modern living because it is under-reported and under-treated. You should be aware that an inability to lose weight and constant fatigue, confusion, or depression could indicate thyroid problems that should be investigated by your doctor.

The Thymus When the thymus gland slows down, the entire immune system is affected. For this reason, the thymus is known as the master gland of the immune system. During the aging process, the thymus can shrink and lose function significantly. Once again, this occurs at an accelerated rate when the HPA axis is in overdrive owing to continually being under a siege of stress. In turn, the immune system becomes inept at fending off infectious invaders as well as at repairing cellular damage. Diseased aging occurs when, owing to a faulty immune system, we break down at a faster rate than we can repair ourselves. Moreover, the immune system begins to mistake as foreign certain substances that naturally occur in the body, attacking and destroying various tissues, glands, and organs. This process is known as autoimmunity; rheumatoid arthritis and lupus are examples of autoimmune disease. Vitamin A, beta carotene, vitamins B6, C, and E, zinc, selenium, and glandular thymus tissue have been shown to help maintain the size and function of the thymus and improve overall immune function.[8]

DIAGRAM 2.1: Neuroendocrine Theory of Aging

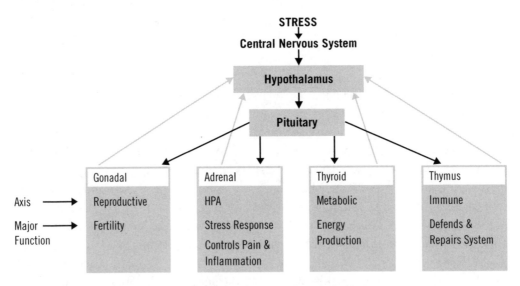

This diagram shows, albeit in a simplified form, how the neuroendocrine system experiences a loss of regulatory function in diseased aging. Stress that is poorly handled—whatever its form or source—overstimulates the hypothalamus. In turn, the hypothalamus (via the pituitary) stimulates the corresponding gland or glands. The solid black arrows issuing from the hypothalamus represent the hypothalamus's action on the four glands, while the grey arrows represent failed attempts by these glands to shut down the hypothalamus. Hypothalamic insensitivity is responsible for glandular failure and diseased aging.

The Pancreas

Poorly regulated blood sugar is the main reason for accelerated and diseased aging. When your blood sugar is well regulated, every biological process in your body functions optimally. The carbohydrates you consume (bread, pasta, cereal, baked goods) are broken down into glucose and cause a rise in blood sugar. The pancreas then secretes insulin to move glucose out of the bloodstream and into important tissues and organs (muscles, liver, heart) to be burned for energy. If you take in too many carbohydrates, especially from refined sources (white bread, white sugar), the pancreas secretes more insulin in an attempt to dispose of this excess glucose.

An Excess of Insulin

If insulin levels are chronically elevated, the cells of your body eventually become resistant to it. Once insulin resistance is established, glucose cannot enter cells to be burned for energy production; this means that blood glucose levels rise. The pancreas perpetuates the problem by pumping more insulin into your system in the hope of getting rid of the glucose that has piled up in your blood.

Chronic high blood levels of insulin (a condition known as *hyperinsulinemia*) cause sugar to be stored as fat, prevent the burning of fat for energy, and cause the liver to over-produce cholesterol. Also, hyperinsulinemia and insulin resistance lead to hypertension, obesity, lipidemia (elevated cholesterol), and diabetes. The members of this quartet are all major risk factors for heart disease and rapid aging. In people with hyperinsulinemia, metabolism comes to a screeching halt, weight gain often occurs, inflammatory processes blaze out of control, and chronic pain and fatigue become the daily grind.

An Excess of Glucose

In some instances of insulin resistance, the pancreas becomes exhausted and can no longer compensate by secreting more insulin. As production of insulin stops, glucose accumulates in the blood. We call this condition diabetes. The excessive glucose gums up all proteins in the body (a process called *glycosylation*), rendering them non-functional and structurally distorted. For instance, when hemoglobin (the oxygen-binding protein in red blood cells) is caked with glucose, the brain, heart, and muscles receive less oxygen. Muscles atrophy, brain function declines, arteries harden, and stroke and heart attack become more likely. Glycosylation also causes connective tissues to stiffen, making your joints inflexible. The skin loses tone and elasticity and becomes wrinkled. When sugar encrusts the lens of the eye, cataracts form and vision becomes cloudy. If this happens to the retina in the eye, blindness sets in. Glycosylation also singes the nerves; hands and feet go numb, making fine motor skills difficult. Sufferers become slow mentally as well; their recall is poor and their thoughts are scattered. And these are just a sample of the changes caused by glucose-encrusted proteins. Clearly, if you want to ensure healthy aging and stave off disease, you must regulate your blood sugar.

Genetic Potential

Our genetic makeup was forged over several hundreds of thousands of years. Today we are learning a great deal about the 23 pairs of chromosomes and the 30,000 or so genes contained in the nucleus of each cell. The collective sum of these genes is known as the human genome, and with great variability it determines our maximum life span.

Some researchers have been seduced by the notion that a single gene might determine longevity or vary the rate of aging or be responsible for age-related diseases. This is an odd expectation, given that rarely have even inherited diseases been found to be the result of mutations in a single gene. Many genes, in fact, are involved in all age-related changes and diseases. And that's good news, since it suggests that much of our physical fate is modifiable. More importantly, we are beginning to understand how diet, lifestyle, and the environment influence the way these genes are expressed, creating either a healthy you or a sick you. Why did Shirechiyo Izumi of Japan live in good health to the age of 120 years and 237 days? Certainly there exists a unique genetic potential for each and every one of us.

Conclusion

One theory, one gene, or the decline of one hormone cannot explain why so many of us are robbed of our genetic potential. The explanation lies in the collection of factors presented in this chapter and summed up here:

- Abuse and overuse of the body
- Exposure to environmental toxins
- Poor detoxification
- Inadequate supply of nutrients
- Inability to control free radicals
- Insufficient energy production
- Poor immune function
- Glandular failure
- Excessive cortisol
- Excessive insulin
- Excessive glucose
- Chronic inflammation
- Physical inactivity
- Excessive caloric intake
- Obesity

These are the factors that make up the pieces of the aging puzzle. Stress is the biggest piece of all, and the smaller pieces are connected to it. Make no mistake, stress—poorly handled and in excessive amounts—is what causes all the health problems discussed in this chapter. Now turn to Chapter 3 to learn more about the things that undermine enduring health.

3

SABOTEURS OF HEALTH

As you read in Chapter 2, many factors affect the aging process, and many of these are under your control. Your goal should not be just to add years to your life, but to add life to your years. You can realize this goal if you take steps to prevent the onset of diseases that cause premature aging and death.

Your body is a well-designed machine that requires care and maintenance; to keep it fine-tuned throughout your long life, you need to understand some of the most serious threats to its smooth performance. Smoking, stress, lack of sleep, poor diet, and inactivity are the greatest saboteurs of health; they can throw a big wrench into the workings of your body, seriously compromising how well you function and how long you'll live. We are now going to examine why and how these saboteurs have a negative impact on health. Don't be discouraged if you are affected by some of them. We will be looking at ways to implement damage control and make positive changes. Knowledge is power!

Up in Smoke

Smoking is the single most preventable cause of death in our society and without a doubt the greatest saboteur of health. In the developed countries, smoking kills over 2 million people each year,[1] and in the United States 430,700 deaths per year are attributable to smoking.[2] Approximately half of all smokers die from diseases caused by smoking, and of these, approximately half die in middle age (35–69), losing an average of 20–25 years of life expectancy.[3]

The adverse health effects of nicotine are numerous. Nicotine affects the hormonal systems, metabolism, and the brain. It is a major cause of heart disease, stroke, and lung disease, and it increases the risk of peptic ulcer, osteoporosis, infection, infertility, sleep disorders, anxiety, and depression. In addition to being responsible for 87 percent of lung cancers, smoking is also associated with cancers of the mouth, pharynx, larynx, esophagus, pancreas, uterine cervix, kidney, and bladder.[4]

Despite all these well-documented health effects, people continue to puff. For those who started years ago, the addiction, habit, pleasure, and social aspects make the practice hard to break. The body has become physically and psychologically dependent on nicotine. But what is truly shocking is the level of smoking among teenagers. A 1999 national survey showed that more than one-third (35 percent) of U.S. high school students were current cigarette smokers (smoked at least one cigarette in the past month).[5]

The Secondhand Effects

You don't have to be a smoker to suffer tobacco's damaging health effects. Secondhand smoke (also called environmental tobacco smoke—ETS) contains numerous human carcinogens for which there is no safe level of exposure. Scientific consensus groups, such as the Environmental Protection Agency, have reviewed the data on ETS:

- Each year about 3,000 nonsmoking adults die from lung cancer as a result of breathing secondhand smoke.
- ETS causes an estimated 35,000 to 40,000 deaths from heart disease in people who are not current smokers.
- ETS causes coughing, phlegm, chest discomfort, and reduced lung function in nonsmokers.
- ETS contains over 4,000 substances, more than 40 of which are known or suspected to cause cancer in humans and animals.

Quit Smoking ... Live Longer

It is never too late to quit smoking, whatever your age. Consider the following facts. One year after quitting, your excess risk of coronary heart disease is half that of a smoker's. Two years after stopping, your risk of lung cancer decreases by about one-third and the risk of heart attack returns to average. Ten years after quitting, your risk of lung cancer returns nearly to normal. After 15 years off cigarettes, your risk of cigarette-associated death returns to nearly the level of those who have never smoked.[6]

There are many options available to help you kick the habit. Gum, patches, oral medication, acupuncture, counseling, and hypnosis are just some of them. Don't be discouraged if you try and fail. It often takes more than one attempt to succeed. Consult with your health practitioner to find the best method for you.

Super Stressed?

Are you living in the fast lane? Are you running around with no time to relax, feeling overwhelmed and burned out? Do you experience racing heart, anxiety, and insomnia? If so, you could be paving your way to *Stressville*. This is a road too many of us follow and it leads us to a place we don't want to be, a place of disease, premature aging, and death.

About 50 years ago, Dr. Hans Selye defined stress as "the non-specific response of the body to any demand placed upon it."[7] In other words, stress is not an external force but rather the body's reaction to external stimuli. It is how we react to rush-hour traffic, to children squabbling, to deadlines at work. Because his patients had similar physiological and psychological characteristics, Dr. Selye recognized the mind–body connection involved with stress. He claimed that it isn't stress that harms us but *distress*. Distress occurs when we prolong emotional stress and don't deal with it in a positive manner.

The Stress Response

In response to stress, the body releases two stress hormones, catecholamines (adrenaline and noradrenaline) and glucocorticoids (cortisol). Secreted by the adrenal glands, these hormones prepare the body to fight; this is the fight-or-flight response. When this occurs, the body enters a catabolic state; that is, it begins to break down fuels (fats, stored sugar) to provide energy. Heart rate, blood pressure, blood volume, and pulmonary (lung) tone increase to enhance the function of the heart and lungs. This innate mechanism was designed to help us cope with short bursts of stress, such as that caused by the attack of a predator. Our bodies have not adapted to handle the chronic stress so common today. This chronic stress thus leads to damage and destruction of the body.

Impact on Health

Stress is associated with many health risks and problems—headaches, insomnia, nervousness, depression, anxiety, skin disorders, musculo-skeletal problems, constipation, diarrhea, weight loss, high blood pressure, exacerbation of asthma, ulcers, arthritis, decreased concentration, panic attacks, colitis, immune deficiency, infertility, reduced sexual drive, and increased risk of cancer. According to the American Psychological Association,

- 43 percent of all adults suffer adverse health effects from stress;
- stress-related ailments and complaints account for 75 to 90 percent of all visits to physicians; and
- stress is linked to the six leading causes of death—heart disease, cancer, lung ailments, accidents, cirrhosis of the liver, and suicide.[8]

The cortisol secreted during stress may help us handle acute physical stressors successfully, but it can have a variety of deleterious effects if secreted chronically and in excess. In excess, cortisol can wreak havoc on the nervous system, particularly the hippocampus, the area of the brain responsible for memory, concentration, and cognitive function. In extreme cases, it can compromise the ability of neurons (nerve cells) to survive stress, and the result is neuron death.

Chronic stress is also implicated in the onset of diabetes. During periods of stress, the body tries to create more energy and glucose levels rise. This triggers the release of insulin, but its effects are blunted by cortisol. The pancreas responds by pumping out more insulin; over time, as the body becomes less sensitive to insulin's effects, insulin resistance occurs. This is a hallmark feature of Type 2 diabetes.

Stress and the Immune System

Have you noticed that you get sick during times of intense stress? This is because stress lowers your lymphocyte (a kind of immune cell) count and increases your body's production of free radicals. Both of these effects weaken the immune system and increase the risk of infection. In fact, the most common causes of weakened immunity in healthy individuals are stress and aging. A 1993 study indicated that the higher the subject's reported level of stress (whether assessed according to negative life-change events, perceived stress level, or the expression of negative feelings), the greater the likelihood that the subject would come down with a cold.[9] The common finding is that a person's chances of developing a physical illness increase with the number of life changes and the amount of stress experienced.

Lack of Sleep

Sleep is one of our most basic needs, for it affects our emotional and physical well-being. Starting the day after a poor night's sleep is like starting out on a long road trip with only a quarter tank of gas. At some point we will run out of fuel. An occasional restless night is no cause for concern, but chronic sleep loss can affect memory and concentration, and lead to depression, headaches, and other maladies. Stress is often a cause of insomnia, but insomnia in turn can cause stress, since it increases the level of hormones, such as cortisol, that cause stress.

Stress can reduce the production of other hormones. According to a recent study, a lack of deep sleep can cause a decline in growth hormone levels.[10] Growth hormone deficiency has been linked to increased obesity, loss of muscle mass, reduced exercise capacity, and accelerated aging. There is no concrete evidence that maintaining higher levels of growth hormone will lengthen your life, but doing so could improve your health.

Sleepless Society

Insomnia can affect anyone, but those over 60 or with a history of depression are at greater risk. A recent poll found that 60 percent of American adults experience sleep problems and that few recognize the importance of adequate rest or are aware of the effective methods of preventing and managing sleep problems now available.[11] Those who had trouble getting enough sleep reported greater difficulty concentrating, accomplishing required tasks, and handling minor irritations.

Lifestyle choices have a huge impact on sleep quality. Excessive caffeine intake during the day, an alcoholic drink before bedtime, lack of exercise, poor diet (too much sugar and processed foods), use of prescription medication, and smoking are some of the biggest culprits. See Chapter 5 for tips on how to develop good sleep hygiene and beat insomnia.

The Erosion of Our Diet

While we all recognize the importance of good nutrition, many of us continue to pollute our bodies with foods and chemicals detrimental to health. The refined grains, excessive sugar, alcohol, caffeine, saturated fat, and trans fatty acids in our diet rob us of essential nutrients, increase our risk of disease and illness, and may cleave years off our lives.

Refined Grains

Refinement is good if we are talking about oil for our cars, but not if we are talking about a process that takes whole grains (such as whole wheat) and turns them into refined flours (white flour). The refining process removes the grain's outer layer of bran and germ, the layer that contains most of the B vitamins, iron, vitamin E, and fiber. The result is a less nutritious, lower-fiber product. Since most North Americans consume only a third of the recommended 25–35 grams of fiber a day, these losses add up.

A high-fiber diet prevents diverticulosis (an intestinal problem), helps lower cholesterol, and offers protection against heart disease and certain cancers. Whole grains don't cause a rapid increase in blood sugar like their refined counterparts. Improved blood-sugar control is particularly important for diabetics and those suffering from hypoglycemia. Even though most flour products now have nutrients added to them (they are "enriched" or "fortified"), health professionals agree that it is better to eat whole grains.

Sugar—Not So Sweet

Would you believe that the average North American consumes 160 pounds of sugar each year? It is true. Four cans of cola daily, each can providing 39 grams (1.375 ounces) of sugar, would alone account for 125 pounds. The obvious sources of sugar are candy, cookies, doughnuts, and ice cream, but most of us don't think about the hidden sources, such as ketchup, peanut butter, and mayonnaise. All these add up to too much sugar and potential health risks.

A diet high in refined sugar has been linked to diabetes, obesity, elevated triglycerides (a type of blood lipid [fat]), tooth decay, poor immune function, and allergies. Overindulging in sweets can affect emotional well-being, causing mood swings, irritability, and anxiety. Moreover, refined sugar contains propyl alcohol, a substance that cannot be broken down in the body; its accumulation in the intestines can disrupt digestion and cause other adverse effects.

Not only is too much sugar bad for you; it also displaces healthier foods in your diet. Take the cola example again: for people on a 2,000-calorie diet, three and a half cans daily would count for 17 percent of their allotted carbohydrates before they've taken in fruits, vegetables, or other essential nutrients.

For better health, avoid refined sugar. If you crave something sweet, have a piece of fruit (fresh or dried). Dried fruits provide concentrated sources of vitamins and minerals along with fiber. Good food sweeteners to consider are honey, maple syrup, malt syrups, and date sugar. These products provide some nutritional value and are not as hard on blood-sugar levels. In baked goods, mashed bananas and apples are a great substitute for sugar. Artificial sweeteners such as aspartame and saccharin should be avoided because they have been linked to headaches, mental illness, brain damage, and cancer. Stevia, a sweetener obtained from a plant from Latin America, appears to be a safe sugar substitute; depending on how it is processed, it can provide up to 300 times the sweetening power of sugar—without the calories.

Trans Fatty Acids

We get several types of fat in our diet, some good, some bad, and some very bad. This continues to be a confusing issue thanks to conflicting reports in the media. A good example is the butter-versus-margarine debate. Butter, an animal product, contains saturated fat, and diets high in saturated fat are linked to high cholesterol, heart disease, cancer, and obesity. Margarine has been thought to be a healthy substitute, but this is not always the case. Margarine is made up of vegetable oils that are hardened by a process called hydrogenation. In this process, the oil becomes less polyunsaturated (more saturated, like butter) and the molecular configuration is altered, creating trans fatty acids.

There is compelling evidence that trans fats are worse than those they were intended to replace; they have a negative impact on blood cholesterol levels and have been linked to heart disease. A recent report linked trans fatty acids and breast cancer, and most disturbing are the studies suggesting that trans fatty acids compromise fetal and infant early development. It's clearly best to pass on the hydrogenated margarines and look for a soft-tub, non-hydrogenated product, such as Becel™. If you like butter, use it sparingly.

Caffeine: No Redeeming Qualities

How do most North Americans jump-start their day? With a cup of coffee, of course. But some of us don't stop there; we have cup after cup, enjoying the aroma and stimulating effects. Coffee drinking has become a social habit and addiction for millions. Some of us get our caffeine jolt from other sources, such as tea, cola, or chocolate. We don't think of caffeine as a drug, yet it has drug-like effects. Pharmacologically, it is classified as a mild stimulant. It "wakes up" the central nervous system, stimulates the digestive tract, speeds up metabolism, and raises brain levels of serotonin, a neurotransmitter that affects mood. In high doses, caffeine can cause rapid heartbeat, irritability, nausea, vomiting, insomnia, and anxiety. Regular consumption can lead to addiction. Abrupt withdrawal, even if you drink only one cup a day, can cause headaches, irritability, and fatigue.

Medical reports have linked caffeine to heart disease, palpitations, certain types of cancer, fibrocystic breast disease, osteoporosis, depression, anxiety, tremors, insomnia, infertility, and other medical problems. Women who are pregnant or are trying to get pregnant, as well as people who experience irregular heartbeats or palpitations, are often advised to cut back on or eliminate caffeine-containing substances.

Moderate caffeine intake (three 8-ounce cups of coffee, or 250 milligrams, per day) is generally not a problem; ten 8-ounce cups of coffee per day is excessive, posing an increased risk of adverse health effects.

Overeating Shortens Life Expectancy

How many of us eat when we're not hungry, try to finish our plate after we're full, eat when we feel sad, or opt for desert after a big meal? Overeating—taking in more calories than our bodies require—is something we commonly do, not thinking of the health consequences. To make matters worse, overeating is encouraged by restaurant chains that offer "Super-Size" and "Biggie" food portions.

Overeating and one of its health consequences—obesity—are known to shave years off your life. Obesity adds stress to the heart, bones, muscles, and other organs, increasing your risk of chronic disease and early death. Researchers believe that overeating also taxes the organs by generating free-radical damage and impeding the body's ability to repair itself. As you age, your basal metabolic rate (the rate at which you burn calories) decreases. This means that if you consume as many calories as you did in your youth, you have a greater chance of gaining weight. Food is also more likely to be converted into fat than into protein and to find its way to your belly and hips.

Scientists have known for years that animals that eat less live longer and suffer fewer age-related diseases. Research in many species, from fruit flies to rats, has shown that a 30 percent caloric restriction can lead to a 30 percent longer life. Dr. Roy Walford conducted some of the pioneering research in this area.[12] Caloric restriction slows metabolism, and since free radicals are by-products of metabolism, caloric restriction may also reduce free-radical damage. Since caloric restriction also lowers body temperature, cells may sustain less genetic damage and repair more readily than at normal body temperature. Scientists also speculate that caloric restriction preserves the cells' capacity to proliferate, moderates the decline in growth hormone, and keeps the immune system functioning at youthful levels.[13] This concept will be covered further in Chapter 7.

A Sobering Look at Alcohol

As a social beverage, alcohol is popular because of its ability to reduce anxiety, tension, and inhibitions. While moderate intake may offer some health benefits, alcohol contributes to 100,000 deaths annually, making it the third leading cause of preventable mortality in the United States, after tobacco and poor diet/activity patterns.[14] More than 7 percent of the adult population drink excessively, a statistic that includes 8.1 million alcoholics.

Alcohol is a central nervous system depressant. Small amounts can slow reactions and impair alertness, concentration, and judgement. Excessive amounts can cause intoxication and poisoning. Alcohol is the single most important cause of illness and death from liver disease (alcoholic hepatitis and cirrhosis). The liver isn't the only site of destruction. Heavy and chronic drinking (more than 3 cups per day) is linked to cardiovascular disease, pancreatitis, immune system depression, increased risk of cancer (esophagus, mouth, liver, breast, and colon), sexual dysfunction (impotence), infertility, and malnutrition. Consumption during pregnancy can afflict the developing fetus with fetal alcohol syndrome.[15]

Alcohol and Brain Aging

According to a recent report, heavy drinking contributes to shrinkage of the frontal lobe of the brain, particularly as individuals age.[16] This area is responsible for emotions, planning, and other higher behavior. Researchers, using a scanning technique called MRI, measured the frontal-lobe volumes of more than 1,400 individuals ranging in age from 30 to 69. Heavy drinkers were nearly twice as likely to experience brain shrinkage as people who didn't drink, while moderate consumption didn't appear to have any effect on the brain. For people aged 30 to 50, heavy drinking doubled the risk that the volume of the brain's frontal lobe would decrease. The good news is that alcoholic brain damage is partly reversible. Individuals who give up the bottle can recover brain volume and boost blood flow. Researchers estimate that aging accounts for about 30 percent of brain shrinkage and heavy alcohol consumption for about 10 percent.

Alcohol—the Good News

In recent years, researchers have found a correlation between moderate alcohol intake and a reduced risk of heart disease. Moderate drinking is defined as no more than one drink a day for women and no more than two for men. Twelve ounces of beer, 5 ounces of wine, or 1.5 ounces of distilled spirits (80 proof) all count as one drink.[17] At least 12 studies have demonstrated that consumption of one or two drinks a day is associated with a 30–50 percent reduced risk of heart disease.[18] Approximately 50 percent of the protective effect of alcohol is related to its ability to increase levels of HDL ("good") cholesterol;[19] the other 50 percent may be attributed to reduced blood-clotting and antioxidant effects, as seen with red wine and dark beer.

Couch Potatoism

Computers, remote control devices, the automobile, and other conveniences have created a lazy society. We can go through our daily routine without exerting ourselves—we drive to work, take the elevator, sit at a computer all day, watch TV at night, and do it all again the next day. And who has time to exercise? Not many of us. According to Canada's National Population Health Survey (1996/97), only 21 percent of people age 12 and over were classified as "sufficiently active" during their leisure time and 57 percent were classified as "inactive." Lack of time and energy are the most common excuses for inactivity offered by the sedentary folk. If you have been leading a sedentary lifestyle, take heed: being inactive increases your risk of developing age-related chronic diseases or conditions like high blood pressure, heart disease, diabetes, obesity, osteoporosis, and cancer. Study after study has demonstrated that if you exercise or are physically active in your daily routine, you can drastically reduce this risk. Exercise also offers mental benefits by reducing stress, anxiety, and depression; improving memory, concentration, and alertness; improving sleep; and boosting self-esteem and self-image. Chapter 6 will give you the tools you need to develop a safe and effective exercise program to meet your needs.

Conclusion

In evaluating your current lifestyle, ask yourself how many of these saboteurs affect you. This chapter should have made it clear that the greatest saboteurs of health are factors you can control. It is all about choices—to quit smoking, to manage your stress level, to get adequate sleep, to have a healthy diet, and to become more physically active. While all this might sound a little overwhelming, it's not so difficult to gradually make the positive changes that will put you on the path to better health. Start making them now, before health problems develop.

4

MEASUREMENTS OF SUCCESSFUL AGING

We will now look at some real stories of older individuals who have successfully aged. These stories reveal the common attributes responsible for a long and successful life. By comparing yourself with these people, you'll be able to measure your physical, psychological, and spiritual dimensions. Just as you need to know your size when shopping for the ideal dress or business suit, you need your measurements for successful aging when you search for a custom-tailored approach that fits you.

The Making of a Legacy

In May 1997 I attended the Fourth International Symposium on Functional Medicine in Aspen, Colorado. I was one of 600 attendees to witness Dr. George Schambaugh receive a special award for his numerous contributions to the field of functional medicine. As Dr. Jeff Bland presented the award to the spry 93-year-old, we all stood and applauded. Dr. Schambaugh's warm smile filled the room as he gracefully accepted the showers of thanks. I remember marveling that a man of his age could still be excited about learning.

George Schambaugh was born on June 30, 1903, and passed away on February 7, 1999. One week before his death, he was still treating patients at the Randolph-Schambaugh Clinic in Illinois. Dr. Schambaugh was a leader in the treatment of allergies, particularly those induced by food and environmental factors. First and foremost he recommended lifestyle and dietary changes to all his patients. His lifelong dedication to the well-being of his patients and his pioneering spirit inspired his colleagues and countless others.

What Makes 100 Worthwhile Years?

There are many like Dr. Schambaugh. Since 1994, the New England Centenarian (NEC) Study has been providing a great deal of information about the intangible elements that 100-year-olds possess.[1] Take 106-year-old James Hanlon, married for 80 years and still living with his 101-year-old wife, Florence. He attributed his vigor and longevity to, among many things, morning leg-lifts and power breakfasts—oatmeal, apples, raisins, and olive oil. Florence insisted that a simple maxim allowed them to live together for so long: "Don't make a federal case out of everything."

Many participants in the study remained active by pursuing their crafts. Edward Fisher, a 102-year-old retired tailor, mended clothes for his fellow residents at the Center for Aged. He also maintained an intimate relationship with one of the female residents. In the interests of medical science, he agreed that on his passing his brain could be examined. Pathologists found Mr. Fisher's brain to be relatively free of plaques and neurological entanglements, often indicative of Alzheimer's and believed to be the normal state of an aging brain. Could it be that Mr. Fisher's involvement and zest for life thwarted the expected in the aging brain?

What can be said about Dirk Struik, a 104-year-old mathematician whose investigations in the field of enthomathematics, publications, and lecturing engagements spanned his lifetime? The contributions he made to tensor calculus when he was a professor at MIT in the 1920s were used by Albert Einstein to prove his theory of relativity. Professor Struik never stopped asking questions, perhaps because his brain saw no limitations.

Equally impressive is the story of Lola Blonder, whose hearing, eyesight, and mind were impeccably intact when she was 101. Mrs. Blonder took up watercolor painting in her nineties, and she was a captivating storyteller. According to researchers who interviewed her, she displayed dignity, energy, imagination, and a warm magnetism. Although slightly physically disabled, she had sacrificed nothing else to time.

Even though Marie Knowles, age 104, never earned more than $7,200 a year, her philosophy of life was rich indeed. Her principles led her to leave an administrative job with the Visiting Nurses Association in Brooklyn, New York. Why? Simply because she felt her fellow nurses were more focused on their pay and pension plans than on their patients. Her life experiences deepened her personal integrity. She felt that having a positive mental attitude and eating sparsely were imperative for long life.

The Maximum So Far

What is longest life ever recorded? Born in Arles, France, on February 21, 1875, Jeanne Louise Calment died at the age of 122 on August 4, 1997. When she made it to 120 years

and 238 days, surpassing the mark set by our Japanese man, Mr. Izumi, she said in explanation, "God must have forgotten me." Jeanne took up fencing at 85 and zipped around
on a bicycle at 100. In the last few years of her life, she was blind, partially deaf, and
confined to a wheelchair, but her spirit still bloomed. "Always keep your smile. That's how
I explain my long life. I think I will die laughing," she once said. She overcame many
things in her life, but vanity was never a hindrance: "I've only ever had one wrinkle and
I'm sitting on it." Clearly her sense of humor afforded her many good years. How did she
die? She died of natural causes in her sleep. Her heart stopped beating.

Necessary Psychological Factors for the Trek to 100

That these centenarians enjoyed good physical and mental health and remained functional for most of their lives demonstrates that becoming old and becoming ill are not the
same thing. Attaining old age for these people was not a process of enduring a long
decline in health but one of avoiding disease altogether. But how did they escape the age-
related diseases that most adults develop between their fifties and nineties? Among many
attributes, it is their psychological approach to life that sets them apart from the pack.

Healthy centenarians have an exuberant spirit that allows them to be productive all
their lives. Rather than withdraw from life as they age, they remain engaged by learning
new things and developing new interests long after their careers end. Whether through
music or art or other activities, they don't stop developing mentally or spiritually. While
they reminisce fondly about the past, they eagerly live in the present and look forward to
the future.

They do not fear death. Humor gives them a perspective about their lives, allowing
them to accept the inevitability of their imminent passing. Joke telling and laughter is a
common feature of these long-lived people. We now know that laughter "exercises" the
heart, thereby improving circulation and oxygenating the entire body. Laughing on a
regular basis improves immune function and stimulates the release of certain neurotransmitters that raise mood and improve mental alertness.

Maintaining their relationships with family and friends is an important priority for
healthy centenarians. When their support network dies, they make new friends and adopt
new people as family. With a social net, they can recover from emotional setbacks and deal
with physical sickness. Indeed, research shows that older people with many friends are far
more likely to survive a heart attack than people with few or no friends. Those with
friends can adapt to all of life's situations with less cortisol (a damaging stress
hormone)—that is, in an efficient and lasting way. They can shed the stress hurled
their way.

Almost all centenarians have a belief in a higher power. Through prayer, attending
church, and partaking in fellowship, they maintain a relationship with God. Many
researchers feel that a relationship with God allows the aged to endure. With God as a

partner, the healthy old are almost never lonely, for they tend to attract loyal people in their lives. Beyond wisdom they have love to offer.

There are indeed many things that help people maneuver their way through life. Three of the most important are a sense of coherence, self-esteem, and mastery. People with a sense of coherence believe that events are comprehensible, challenges are manageable or will pass, and life is meaningful. Those with self-esteem evaluate their own attributes positively and have a sense of worth as an individual. People with a sense of mastery feel that they have control over what happens to them and the ability to resist negative influences; in sum, mastery is the ability to be the producer, director, and actor in your own motion picture.

This trio helps you deal with conflict successfully and in turn permits feelings of contentment and wholeness. People don't grow when they fail to come to terms with life. Such a failing may very well open the door to disease. To grow old and stay healthy, you must continue to grow mentally, psychologically, emotionally, and spiritually. Thomas T. Perls, Margery Hutter Silver, and John F. Lauerman summed this up in their book *Living to 100:*

> *A profound peacefulness prevails: centenarians are ready for death but still engaged in life. They no longer think about past mistakes or losses, nor do they struggle to integrate the contradictions and ambivalences of their long lives. They don't ruminate about whether or not their lives had meaning—they are still actively finding meaning in their lives. They warm quickly to telling stories about their struggles and successes of the past, and often perceive and portray themselves as crucial characters in the events that unfold around them.*[2]

Life can be sweet but only if you choose it to be. The New England Centenarian Study and many others as well[3] have suggested a number of the intangible elements of healthy longevity:

- The ability to attract people
- An ability to be assertive
- An ability to express feelings
- An ability to experience joy, happiness, and love
- An ability to give direction to your life
- A commitment to grow psychologically and spiritually
- A positive mental attitude
- A sense of purpose
- A sense of confidence and trust in self
- A strong connection to family, community, and God
- A sense of humor
- A sense of peace, acceptance of mortality

- A willingness to learn
- A willingness to overcome upsets and disappointments

A Matter of Attitude

People who have a pessimistic outlook and worry excessively are overwhelmed by the small things. Constant anxiety and fear can flood the body with all sorts of stress chemicals that eventually break it down bit by bit. While these chemicals help us deal with confrontation, we will inevitably incur damage if we see every situation as a battle. Researchers have pointed out that this type of emotional stress accelerates aging and causes the hippocampus—the part of the brain responsible for memory, mood, and drive—to shrink.[4] Your rate of aging isn't determined so much by the amount of stress you deal with as by how you respond to stress.[5] Know that your mental attitude influences how you'll behave under stress.

What about Weight?

There are physical attributes that increase functional span and postpone the disability zone. One study showed that 99 percent of its participants 100 years of age and older did not meet the criteria for obesity. In fact, the current weight of almost 80 percent of the centenarians was close to the weight they maintained throughout their entire lives by eating moderately and sensibly.[6] Remember, avoiding obesity greatly reduces the risk of heart disease, hypertension, diabetes, and most types of cancer. Thus, maintaining ideal body weight is a must for those wanting to trek to 100.

Calculating Your Body Mass Index

An important biological marker, body mass index (BMI), correlates well with fat-free mass and a person's overall body composition. BMI is an acceptable range of weight in proportion to your height. The BMI is calculated as follows:

$$BMI = \frac{Weight\ (kg)}{Height\ (m^2)} \quad or \quad BMI = \frac{Weight\ (lb.) \times 705}{Height\ (in.^2)}$$

An acceptable BMI for men is from 20.7 to 26.4; for women it is anywhere from 19.1 to 25.8. A BMI under or over these values is an indication that weight needs to be gained or lost, and those changes need to occur in body composition. Bodybuilders are an exception; typically they have low body fat but often a slightly higher than expected BMI, since muscle weighs more than fat. These individuals are not believed to be at any greater risk of developing obesity-related diseases.

Spirits for the Soul

We have all heard the "business" about drinking a daily glass of red wine to avoid heart disease. Most centenarians, however, don't consume alcohol on a daily basis. In fact, it is hard to find a history of alcoholism among centenarians. When these people did consume alcohol, it was done sensibly. Being sensible seems to be the common approach to most things among centenarians. And when it comes to smoking, it's virtually nonexistent in the lives of centenarians. The few who did smoke did so for only a short period early in their lives.

Exercising Mind and Body

Mentally exerting the brain through crossword puzzles, reading and writing, learning new things, and problem solving helps to keep it sharp. The brain actually grows by use! And this occurs at any age. Even if there's been prior damage caused by, say, a stroke, the brain can be "rewired" to form new connections, bypassing the area of injury and thus compensating for any loss of function.

When brain function is maintained, the "executive" function (the ability to plan, organize, and complete a task) can be kept operational. Your brain's executive function will influence how well you'll maintain your independence in old age. Follow the example of our enviable centenarians and find enjoyable ways to exercise your mind.

Being physically active was another part of the repertoire for the healthy old throughout their entire lives. At 102 Tom Spears could play 18 holes of golf three times a week, providing a new yardstick for being in shape. How about Anna Morgan, who at 101 engaged her mind by reading while riding a stationary bike? Also 101, William Cohen still owned a printing business and worked there several days a week. In fact, all the centenarians in the New England study had a full day's activity on their agenda each and every day.

A routine of strength and weight-bearing exercises helps you avoid loss of muscle and bone mass. Regular exercise also strengthens the heart muscle, thereby improving circulation and keeping blood pressure and heart rate well regulated. Moreover, exercising helps increase basal metabolic rate (this will be described below) and keeps blood cholesterol and body fat in check. Aerobic capacity is also improved by exercising. If you're 55 and can't go up a flight of stairs without huffing and puffing, you are out of shape because of a very low aerobic capacity.

An immediate effect of regular exercise is a new sense of confidence in dealing with stress; this in turn bolsters self-esteem. Physically active individuals are calmer, in better and more stable moods, and less plagued by bouts of depression than their sedentary opposites. In coming chapters we will discuss how you can start and maintain a regular exercise program. Getting off the couch will help you avoid the risk of age-related diseases and will enhance your chances of attaining a maximum functional life span.

Measuring Your True Age

Chronological age represents the actual number of years, months, and days that have elapsed since you were born. It does not, however, give us a complete picture of your body's true age or the rate at which aging is taking place. Biological age gives us a better idea of your true age. Our healthy centenarians had the biology and resiliency of youth. They were devoid of virtually all age-related diseases, were cognitively intact and emotionally stable, and had warm personalities. Clearly, their biological age was much lower than their chronological age.

Determinants of Biological Age

Biological age is an indication of how well a person is functioning on a physiological level. For instance, the aerobic capacity of people who do not exercise declines by about 10 percent each decade after age 30. Those who engage in moderate exercise can reduce this decline by one-half. Vigorous exercisers typically experience very little decline in aerobic capacity until their sixties, and then it's a modest decline. Your aerobic capacity is a good indicator of biological age.

Basal metabolic rate (BMR) is another indicator of biological age. A person's BMR represents his or her ability to readily burn enough calories to sustain vital bodily functions while at rest. The less muscle mass and the more fat, the lower the BMR. People who don't exercise will typically have their BMR drop by 5 percent (they will burn 100 fewer calories daily) for every decade that flies by. A declining BMR means age-related weight gain. Further, a plummeting BMR means that less energy is being generated to sustain vital bodily functions. All this translates into a higher rate of biological decline. An improved BMR can only be obtained through regular exercise.

Maintaining a lean body (reducing the percentage of body fat and increasing muscle mass) also revs up your BMR. Twenty percent of the weight of the average 25-year-old male is pure fat; the figure is 24 percent for females. By the time 80 years have rolled along, females can expect to have 44 percent body fat, males about 40 percent. The more muscle mass you have, the more calories you burn and the more energy is available to run the vital functions of the body. When muscles are not properly trained, people can lose an average of seven pounds of muscle mass for every passing decade after young adulthood. Muscles are built and maintained only through weightlifting and resistance training. Like the brain, they grow by use—at any age!

The Value of Laboratory Tests

The most easily monitored markers of healthy aging are blood pressure, total cholesterol to HDL ratio, bone density, and blood glucose tolerance. This quartet can be strongly influenced by one's body composition (fat-free mass and aerobic capacity).

As people age, they are more likely to develop high blood pressure. High blood pressure often has no symptoms, and left unchecked, it can lead to heart attack, stroke, kidney damage, and blindness. It is extremely important to have your blood pressure measured on a yearly basis as you age. A normal reading is 140 over 90 and under. Any reading higher than 140 over 90 is considered to be high.

The major reasons for high blood pressure during aging are the loss of elasticity in the circulatory system and the accumulation of oxidized cholesterol, causing the arteries to harden and become blocked. When blood flow is restricted, the heart has to work harder to pump the same amount of blood; this ultimately increases the pressure in the entire cardiovascular system. There are two types of cholesterol, and it is important to understand the difference. High-density lipoprotein (HDL) is known as the "good cholesterol"; low-density lipoprotein (LDL) as the "bad cholesterol." HDL protects the cardiovascular system by removing excess cholesterol and bringing it to the liver for disposal. A very high LDL and low HDL reading spells a disaster waiting to happen—thus the great importance of measuring the ratio of LDL to HDL as you get older.

While loss of bone density is another major concern, the biggest landmine to be sidestepped is rising glucose and/or insulin levels. Elevated glucose can lead to diabetes and its related complications. (See Chapter 19.) High insulin levels eventually lead to insulin resistance and virtually all age-related diseases. What's more, your overall functional health is dependent upon well-controlled blood glucose levels with minimal elevations in insulin to accomplish this. That's why blood glucose and insulin levels together comprise the kahuna of all biological markers.

Conclusion

Distilled down, your biological age is your functional age. No, you cannot stop time, and yes, chronologically you will get older. However, your biological function can be optimized and maintained to keep you functional. The appendices relating to this chapter will help you do this. Appendix 4.1 presents a practical list of biomarkers that you can track on a yearly basis to give you an idea of the rate at which aging is taking place. The questionnaire in Appendix 4.2 will give you an idea of your biological age. These appendices will help you find the areas in your life and body that need to be addressed if you expect smooth sailing to 100 and beyond.

PART 2

HEALTH
PRIORITIES

5

CREATING EMOTIONAL BALANCE

Many of us try to do more each day than we did the day before. We strive for greater wealth and more possessions. With more information available to us, we have to learn more and do more at work. Change comes as quickly as the turning pages of the calendar.

This lifestyle comes at a cost. Many succumb to the pressures of stress, anxiety, and depression, losing control of where they are going and what they are doing. We have catchy names for conditions like these: road rage, anxiety attacks, job strain, and burnout. Almost everyone is affected by the growing complexity of our society, some more than others. There are ways to cope with the stressors accompanying the whirlwinds of our days; these coping methods can turn potentially negative stress into positive stress and allow us to enjoy the benefits of our surroundings in good health.

Roughly a third of Canadians report experiencing high levels of personal stress, 35 percent of women and 28 percent of men.[1] Through the 1990s, the levels of stress related to work and family increased significantly. The obligation to sacrifice family time for work or work time for family creates stress for many. In 2001, 59 percent of Canadians felt highly overloaded in their workplace (compared with 47 percent in 1991), and nearly 62 percent felt that their work interfered in their family lives at a medium or high level.[2]

Clinical depression, also known as major depressive disorder, is one of the most common forms of mental illness in North America, affecting approximately 9.9 million Americans every year.[3] The chances of experiencing clinical depression are twice as high for women as for men; at some point in their lives, 5 percent of men and 10 percent of women will suffer clinical depression.[4]

Stress-related problems often manifest themselves as physical health problems. Stress, anxiety, and depression are linked to a number of other factors in overall health. As indicated in Chapter 3, high stress levels can result in chronic health problems that contribute to the six leading causes of death.[5]

The Anatomy of Stress

According to Dr. Hans Selye, the physical experience of continuous stress has three stages: alarm, resistance, and exhaustion. In the alarm stage, our bodies engage in their biologically programmed fight-or-flight mode. Stress hormones are released into our bodies and we become excited, experiencing heightened senses, a faster heartbeat, and increased blood-sugar levels. At this stage, the hypothalamus, the master gland of the endocrine system, receives a strong dose of cortisol from the adrenal glands. At the resistance stage, the body works to heal itself by adapting resistance mechanisms to counter the negative effects of stress. If the stress continues, we may eventually fall into the exhaustion stage. Mental and physical fatigue sets in, and stress-related disorders (headache, nagging pain, insomnia) may surface.

Chronic stress (continuous stress) and regular bouts of acute stress (intense bursts of stress) accelerate the aging process. The hormonal and chemical effects of stress on the body can cause the brain, heart, and other organs to degenerate faster. Links drawn between stress and cancer suggest that increased stress levels lead to a weaker immune system and a higher susceptibility to cancer and cancer growth.

A Positive Attitude

A merry heart doeth good like a medicine: but a broken spirit drieth the bones.
PROVERBS 17: 22

One of the best ways to combat the negative effects of stress is to have, or develop, a positive attitude. More and more scientific research is pointing to the health benefits to be had by dealing with stress properly and maintaining a positive attitude. According to one research study, people with an optimistic approach to life were half as likely to suffer a heart-related event as those with a grimmer view.[6]

The well-publicized Nun Study drew similar conclusions about the relationship between a positive outlook and good mental and physical health. Dr. David Snowdon, a leading expert on Alzheimer's disease, worked with the School Sisters of Notre Dame to explore the relationship between Alzheimer's and various lifestyle factors. In 2001 he published some breakthrough results in his book *Aging with Grace*. His research findings suggested that people who mentally challenge themselves throughout their lives are better able to avoid the debilitating effects of Alzheimer's and that those who maintain a positive outlook live longer.[7]

Maintaining a positive outlook on life, coping with stress, and finding a proper emotional balance are interrelated. People with a positive attitude are more likely to handle stress well. Those who have a negative attitude and don't deal well with stress run the risk of experiencing the exhaustion stage of stress.

The Path to Positivity

The first step along the path to positivity is to take an honest look at yourself. Are you an intense Type-A personality, a worrier, or a people pleaser? Do you view life as a series of successes and failures rather than as a series of learning experiences? What stressors affect you most seriously?

Though you may be a negative thinker in some aspects of your life—we all are to one degree or another—you can turn those negative attitudes into positive ones with a "stay positive" action plan. It is within your power to choose how to respond to different stressors in life. Make a conscious effort to respond positively.

- Treat problems as challenges to be met or puzzles to be solved. A problem can be a learning experience. Focus on finding the best solution. Once you've chosen a solution, create a step-by-step approach to achieve it.
- Recognize that times of trouble are not permanent. Reflect on other tough times and remember how you made it through them. Consider how you grew from those experiences and how the present experience might help you grow as well.
- Keep a proper perspective. There are always people with bigger problems and in worse situations than yours. While this thought may not make you feel better, it should help you feel thankful for what you do have.
- Don't worry about things you can't control. Try to keep your immediate situation in line with your long-term goals and with the things that are most important to you.
- Be aware of your faults and accept them. If you are working with a group, match yourself with someone whose strengths compensate for your weaknesses. If you want to change a personal habit or characteristic, do so in small steps. Don't set yourself up for disappointment by trying to make an abrupt personal change.
- Learn from your mistakes; don't dwell on them. Look for ways to avoid repeating the same mistakes.
- Speak to yourself in a positive manner. As Max Ehrmann wrote in his famous 1927 poem, "Desiderata," "Beyond a wholesome discipline, be gentle with yourself."
- Create personal goals, big and small. Goals provide a sense of direction and focus. The frequent achievement of minor goals will boost your self-esteem and give you a sense of progress.

Dealing with Stress

Coping with stress is a crucial step in developing a positive attitude. Effective coping strategies help prevent stress's deleterious effect on your well-being and the length of your life. Identify the stressors that you respond to negatively, and figure out how to change your reaction or remove yourself from those situations. If you're frustrated by heavy traffic on the way home from work, investigate the possibility of changing your work hours. Or go to the gym after work and leave for home later. Recognize that there are things you can do to limit your exposure to negative stressors. While you may not be able to avoid them, knowing the source of your stress will help you feel more in control. Next, learn effective ways to relieve and minimize your stress. There are many options to consider.

- *Exercise.* Exercise is one of the most effective ways of coping with stress, as it releases nervous energy and induces a calming effect.
- *Massage.* Stress often manifests itself as tension in the muscles and soft tissues, restricting blood and oxygen flow to those areas. A registered therapist can loosen the muscles and improve circulation, filtering out the negative chemical effects of stress.
- *Substance avoidance.* Drugs, such as alcohol, tobacco, and tranquilizers, offer short-term fixes for stress but can worsen the problem over time, causing addiction and side effects such as loss of short-term memory, dizziness, drowsiness, dry mouth, and loss of balance. While many people think that smoking relieves stress and promotes relaxation, recent studies suggest the contrary. In a 1999 study, nicotine dependency was shown to increase stress.[8] Researchers found that regular smokers experience heightened stress and negative moods between cigarettes. While smoking restores stress level to normal, the smoker soon needs another cigarette to prevent the withdrawal symptoms. Smoking and nicotine dependency are thus the cause—not the reliever—of stress. Another reason to kick the habit!
- *Healthy eating.* Fuel your body with a healthy breakfast and lunch to ensure you have the energy to cope with the possibility of unexpected stress.
- *Friendships.* Studies show that close friendships contribute to a longer life. Researchers suspect that the comfort, companionship, and laughter associated with friendships reduce stress, and this translates into improved longevity. If you haven't already, create a network of close friends and spend time with them. Rely on your friends. Don't keep your frustrations to yourself; if you do, your body will absorb the stress that negative emotions create.
- *Balancing home and work.* Develop ways to leave your work problems behind when you come home (and vice versa). If you can compartmentalize these aspects of your life to some degree, you will be able to minimize the stress they cause. Time-management and organizational skills at work and at home are keys to stress reduction. By developing plans and establishing routines, daily challenges are easier to

overcome. Lists and goals can help you prioritize. Check things off as you go and recognize what is most important to you. Don't be inflexible, though; inflexibility can lead to added stress when an unforeseen situation interferes with your plans.

- *Breathing.* Long deep breaths in stressful situations can calm your body, help you relax, and give your body the oxygen it needs to resist the effects of stress properly. Deep breathing triggers what Harvard professor Herbert Benson coined "the relaxation response," a state in which the heart rate slows, blood pressure drops, and muscles relax (responses opposite to those created by stress).
- *Time-out.* Stress can take over your life, so try to remove yourself from stressful situations by taking short, frequent breaks. Just looking out the window for a minute can clear your mind. A small break will calm you down and you'll be more productive when you return to your task. Longer breaks for reflection can help you prepare for what's ahead.
- *Emotional control.* Anger and hostility have been linked to above-average blood cholesterol levels and an increased incidence of heart trouble. Learn to manage anger and frustration. You can choose how to react to a situation; practice controlling or redirecting your anger into something positive.

Stress is the way our bodies react when there is more happening than we can cope with. Recognize what tasks and responsibilities give you stress, and work out the best method for turning down additional commitments when you are in these situations. Make a firm commitment to yourself. Also, learn how to delegate tasks to those who have more time or expertise, spreading the load and—if all goes well—reducing everyone's level of stress. Even when no one else can do the task, don't be afraid to just say no.

Sleep

Sleep is a critical coping defense against stress. Although mysteries remain about what happens to the body during sleep, it is believed that our bodies use this downtime to repair and regenerate. Our sleep–wake patterns are governed by circadian rhythms that develop shortly after birth. In this cycle, there are two natural daily peak times for sleeping, nighttime and midday (siesta time!). The onset of sleep is largely regulated by changes in light and certain hormones produced in the body.

Not everyone requires the same amount of sleep to wake up feeling well rested and energetic, but we all need to find the time for restful sleep. If we don't give our bodies time to recover from stress, we limit the healing opportunity offered by the resistance stage of stress and move closer to the exhaustion stage, where we are mentally and physically less able to handle stress.

Spirituality, Prayer, and Inner Peace

Dozens of studies have suggested that there is a direct link between spiritual/religious beliefs and better health. Spiritually active people live longer and healthier lives, recover from illnesses faster, and cope with stress better, making them less likely to suffer from depression, high blood pressure, heart problems, and other stress-related conditions.[9]

Dr. Benson, the same person who identified "the relaxation response" mentioned above, also developed the theory of "the faith factor." Benson observed that 80 percent of his patients used prayer to elicit a relaxation response and, of that number, 25 percent reported feeling more spiritual afterward.[10] In prayer, these latter triggered the relaxation response, relieving their stress and finding a heightened sense of well-being at the same time.

For some, spirituality and inner peace is achieved through religion and prayer. For others, it involves music, meditation, or yoga. For still others, spirituality is experienced by walking in the woods. For all, spirituality is a means of achieving inner peace, that calming sense of hope and well-being that is so effective in dealing with stress.

The results of a study involving seriously ill people suggested that those who lose their faith experience greater health deterioration than those with a strong faith. Nearly 600 people, age 55 years or older, who were hospitalized in Durham, North Carolina, in 1996 and 1997 were tracked over a two-year period. Those who questioned their faith, felt abandoned by God, or otherwise expressed a weakening in their spiritual beliefs were as much as 28 percent more likely to die within two years.[11]

As a form of prayer or as an exercise on its own, meditation is a great stress-reduction method. It helps you find deep comfort, stillness, and peace within yourself, allowing you to avoid stress despite today's frenetic pace. Meditation makes it easier for you to cope with difficult situations and maintain a positive outlook.

Conclusion

No matter what methods you use, it's important that you create emotional balance in your life. Over time, stress can cripple you, mentally and physically, and nothing overcomes the negative effects of stress better than a positive attitude. Plan to stay on the path to positivity. Figure out which methods of stress control work best for you. Recognize the benefits of sleep. And take the time to find inner peace in whatever fashion you prefer.

The world is likely to continue spinning faster as you move through your life, and that fast pace is inevitably going to cause you stress. By choosing the path to positivity and creating emotional balance, you increase your chances of having a long, active, and healthy life.

6

EXERCISING YOUR WAY TO A YOUNGER BODY

If your life plan is to live each day with energy, freedom of movement, and the ability to live independently, then you should make exercise a priority. Regular exercise decreases the chances of disease and illness and also allows your body to remain strong, flexible, and able to respond to the physical demands of everyday life. A healthy body will carry you further and more easily through life. It will also make the journey enjoyable.

Beginning an exercise program can be overwhelming, especially if you haven't exercised before. If you are wondering where to start and what you should be doing, you are not alone. In this chapter, we hope to clear up the confusion by giving you the tools required to incorporate cardiovascular exercise, muscle conditioning, and flexibility movement into your lifestyle. We also hope to motivate you to begin planning your own exercise program!

The advantages of an active lifestyle range from improved heart and lung function to better sleep patterns, from stronger muscles and bones to an overall healthier outlook on life. Exercising will not only keep your body strong and healthy; it will also help you to deal with life's inevitable mental and emotional stressors.

Beating Obstacles to Exercise

An amazing 80 percent of people don't exercise on a regular basis.[1] Here are some of the more common of an endless number of excuses:

"I don't have enough time."

This is the number one excuse for most people. In reality, it's usually more a matter of a perception of a lack of time than a true inability to fit exercise into the day. When life gets hectic, exercise is the first thing to be dropped from the daily agenda—and it should be the last. Exercise is what is going to keep you sane when the walls of life start squeezing in on you! Look at it this way: your family, your job, and your social life will always be there, but by putting your own needs second, you may end up wondering what happened to your health in the process. Taking care of yourself now means not relying on someone else to take care of you later. Some of the following suggestions might work for you:

- *Make exercise appointments with yourself.* Mark them down so that when you're asked to do something at that time, you can honestly say that you have an appointment.
- *Write down what you do all day.* It's surprising how many "time wasters" creep into a day (TV, the computer). Determine what yours are and work on eliminating them.
- *Fit in some exercise throughout the day.* Wake up 30 minutes earlier and go for a bike ride, walk during lunch hour, take 15-minute stretch breaks, play actively with your children or grandchildren, or do some gardening.
- People who exercise are more productive than those who don't. This means that the better shape you're in, the more you'll accomplish in a day. So, start planning to fit in some movement!

"I have no energy."

A poor excuse, since exercise can actually give you energy. But don't wait till the end of the day when you're tired; instead, schedule your fitness activities for the morning. If you're not an early riser, try to work out right after work. Keep your fitness gear in the car so that you won't have to go home first and see that comfy-looking couch.

"I don't like exercise."

Beginning an exercise program can seem like a chore or punishment. The key is to find activities you enjoy. That way you're more likely to stick to them. Once you feel the physical and mental health benefits of your program, you'll probably find yourself wanting more exercise sessions rather than fewer. Experiencing pain while exercising means you may be overdoing it. The old adage "No pain, no gain" is out the window. If it hurts, don't do it. Keep that in mind and you'll find that exercise can be extremely enjoyable.

"I have stiff joints (or arthritis)."

If you have stiff joints and/or arthritis, it is even more important that you exercise. Stiff joints that aren't moved will become stiffer, less mobile, and more painful, further limiting what you can do in a day. A recent study found that regular exercise may allow older adults suffering from knee osteoarthritis a better quality of life. The study determined that both resistance and aerobic exercise improved the subjects' ability to perform everyday activities important for independent living. Participants reported a decrease in knee pain since they had become active.[2]

"I'm too old."

How about, you are too old *not* to exercise! As you age, your body naturally begins to lose endurance capacity, muscle mass, bone density, and flexibility, especially if you are sedentary. The good news from recent studies is that it is never too late to reap the benefits of regular exercise. In a study involving 80- and 90-year-old nursing home residents, leg muscle strength was increased by 174 percent and muscle size by 9 percent after only eight weeks of weightlifting exercise.[3] Other research has shown that weight training can improve walking speeds, mobility, and independence in daily activities, and reduce dependence on canes, walkers, and wheelchairs. Some research participants almost immediately felt healthier and able to move more freely. In fact, more active older adults have the fitness and function of people much younger.[4] So remember, exercise is a powerful anti-aging tool that can benefit everyone. It is not just for the young and fit!

Now that you've seen the weakness of those anti-exercise excuses, you may be ready to get started. The following sections are going to help you design a program that suits you.

Get Up and Go! Cardiovascular Exercise

Cardiovascular exercise is any form of activity that uses large muscle groups and is carried out for more than a few minutes. With this type of exercise you will usually feel warm and notice that your breathing becomes deeper. Some good examples are walking, cycling, hiking, swimming, dancing, stair climbing, and cross-country skiing.

Cardiovascular exercise strengthens your heart and lungs, improves circulation and breathing patterns, and decreases risk of heart disease, high blood pressure, and stroke. Other benefits include decreased or maintained body weight, increased energy, stronger muscles and bones, mood regulation, improved sleep patterns and digestion, and an overall feeling of better health. You will have more stamina to work and more endurance to play!

"How do I get started?"

Set aside some time for cardiovascular activities you enjoy— a walk each evening, a fitness class at your local recreation center, or a bike ride before work. Things like these are "structured" activities because you plan ahead and make time for them. Another option is to include some "unstructured" activities into your day. Try walking to the store rather than driving, taking the stairs instead of the elevator, or parking your car at the far end of the parking lot at the mall. Unstructured activities are squeezed into your daily routine and don't disrupt your everyday actions. Structured activities take a bit more planning. It's beneficial to do both. You can do unstructured activities on a daily basis and plan to do structured activities (you might call them "exercise sessions") three to seven days a week.

"How long do I have to keep moving?"

Remember: any amount of activity is better than none at all. Still, to gain the greatest benefit from your efforts, you should accumulate 20–60 minutes of endurance exercise over the course of your day. If you can, try moving continuously for the recommended amount of time. If this is too much for you, then break it up. For instance, you might walk for 10 minutes in the morning, another 10 at lunch, and another 10 after dinner. By the end of the day you will have accumulated 30 minutes! As your endurance improves, you will eventually be able to keep going for 20–60 minutes without stopping.

"How hard should I be exercising?"

You need to work in order to benefit, but you don't want to overdo it in the process. The Rating of Perceived Exertion is a good tool to use when embarking on a cardiovascular exercise program.

The Rating of Perceived Exertion (RPE) Scale

This scale monitors your exercise intensity. It is based solely on how you feel while moving. Ask yourself, "How do I feel?" or "How hard is this activity?" Your perception of how hard you are working will indicate whether you are in the appropriate training zone.

In using the RPE Scale, you rate yourself within a range of 0–10, with zero being how you would feel at complete rest (no exertion) and 10 being severe exhaustion (maximal exertion). Since you are the best judge of how you feel, the chance of rating yourself improperly is basically nil.

A good recommendation for the average person is an RPE of 4 to 6. Within this range, you are working hard enough to benefit from your program, but are in no danger of overdoing it and risking injury.

Safety Tips for Cardiovascular Exercise

It's always good to think about safety. You don't want to injure yourself; that would defeat the original purpose of exercising, which was to move you forward on the path to better health and a stronger body. Here are some useful tips:

- Talk with your health-care provider before beginning.
- Always warm up. Begin slow, and then gradually make it more challenging. Give yourself about five minutes of light movement before bumping up the intensity.
- As your endurance builds, progress to more challenging activities.
- Choose activities that you enjoy and can perform comfortably.
- Use comfortable footwear that supports your feet and ankles, preferably something that has been made for exercising. Footwear that laces up or has Velcro straps is preferable to slip-on shoes, as these can slip off while you're exercising.
- Wear comfortable clothing that allows your body to breathe. Dress in layers so that you can always take off or add a layer when needed.
- Drink water to prevent dehydration. Recent recommendations advise that you drink at least 2 cups (500 milliliters) of fluid two hours before exercising and another 2 cups (500 milliliters) approximately 15 to 20 minutes before you begin. While engaged in the activity, you should replenish fluid every 15 to 20 minutes.[5] A good way to determine whether you should be drinking more water is to weigh yourself before and after you exercise. For every pound lost, you should drink 2 cups of water (500 milliliters). These guidelines will help you balance your fluids before, during, and after exercise.
- Stretch after your exercise session to help your muscles relax and recover (see the section on stretching later in this chapter).

Pump Yourself Up!
Muscle Strength and Endurance Activities

Activities that involve muscular strength and endurance challenge your muscles against a resistance. This resistance can be hand weights, rubber tubing, bags of groceries, your own body weight, weight-training machines, full garbage bags, furniture, water, weighted balls, and laundry baskets (to name a few!).

Working against a resistance promotes stronger muscles and bones, helps maintain the bone and muscle mass you already have, and helps to improve your posture and balance. Other benefits include a decreased risk of injury while doing everyday activities, improved muscle tone, and a decreased chance of falling.

"How do I get started?"

First of all, decide where you would like to do your resistance training. You could join a gym or do your exercises at home. A gym offers access to a variety of equipment—weight machines, free weights, exercise balls, rubber tubing, and so on. If you would rather exercise at home, then you have to figure out what you are going to use for resistance. You might buy some hand weights or rubber tubing, use your own body weight, or use household items as your "weights"—soup cans, books, or anything that you can hold comfortably and is heavy enough to provide some resistance.

When you regularly take time out of your day to lift, push, or pull an object, you are creating "structured" exercise. It is recommended that you do structured resistance training two to four days each week. Everyday duties like carrying groceries, moving furniture, digging in the garden, and climbing stairs also challenge your muscles; these are "unstructured" exercises, the routine activities of daily living. You should engage in as many of these unstructured activities as you can.

"How long do I have to challenge my muscles?"

Many sports authorities agree that you need to do one set of 8–12 repetitions of an exercise. If you are over 50, it is recommended that you do 10–15 repetitions in each set. A repetition, or "rep," is a single movement or exercise done several times consecutively. A set is a series of repetitions. For instance, you might do three sets of 12 repetitions each.[6]

A well-rounded program may take anywhere from 15 to 60 minutes. You should choose an exercise for each major muscle group in your body. This means exercises for your upper body, your lower body, and your midsection. Our top picks for these areas are push-ups (wall or floor), squats or mini-squats, abdominal crunches, lunges, and lower-back-strengthening movements. When you're just beginning, it's best to work with a fitness professional to develop a balanced routine.

"How hard do I have to work?"

Use a resistance that causes your muscles momentary fatigue within the recommended number of reps. Momentary fatigue is the point at which you can't do another repetition without losing proper form.[7] If you find that the resistance doesn't tire out your muscles within the recommended reps, try increasing the resistance the next time you exercise (use a heavier weight, heavier book, thicker rubber tubing, etc.). Keep in mind that you should never work to muscle failure. If your muscles are too tired to execute the movement with control and proper technique, it's time to stop.

Safety Tips for Muscular Strength and Endurance Exercise

As we emphasized earlier, it's important to be aware of safety factors before beginning your program:

- Talk to your health-care provider before starting.
- Warm up! A trip up and down your stairs or a short walk around your house will ensure that your muscles are warmed up and ready to handle the upcoming exercises.
- Learn proper technique to protect your joints; try to avoid jerky movements. You should feel in control of the resistance and able to perform the exercise smoothly.
- Build up gradually. Challenge your muscles, but don't overexert them.
- Breathe! Avoid holding your breath. Let yourself breathe naturally. Try exhaling as you exert and inhaling on the recovery part of the movement.
- Don't move your joints past their natural range.
- You should not be in pain. Feelings of fatigue or exertion are normal, but anything you would describe as a sharp, shooting or a dull, grinding pain is a warning signal from your body. Discontinue the exercise if you experience either of these.
- Use the Two-Hour Rule. If within two hours after an exercise session you feel abnormal joint or muscle pain, you need to cut back on your training intensity.[8]
- Be sure to stretch after your exercise session.

Stretch It Out! Flexibility Activities

Flexibility activities promote freedom of movement in your joints by stretching or elongating your muscles. Stretching your muscles every day helps you move more easily, keeps your joints healthy, and maintains your mobility as you age. Other benefits include improved posture, decreased muscle tension, and decreased risk of injury. These activities will also relax you, easing stress. Stretch-and-hold movements, yoga, and Tai Chi are examples of "structured" flexibility exercises; gardening, yard work, and housework are of the "unstructured" variety.

"How do I get started?"

You should stretch every day. You can take time out in the morning, afternoon, or evening, whenever it's most convenient for you. If you can't find time to do all your stretches at once, do a few stretches here and there throughout the day, such as when you're on the phone, watching television, or reading a book. You can also join a yoga or Tai Chi class.

"How long should I stretch?"

Stretches should be held for 10–60 seconds. Holding a stretch for 10 seconds will maintain the flexibility level you have right now. This type of stretching is beneficial after cardiovascular and muscular strength and endurance activities, as it relaxes your muscles after they have been working. To become more flexible than you are now, you should hold your stretches for 30–60 seconds. This will promote elongation of the muscle and allow it sufficient time to respond to the movement.

"How should a stretch feel?"

Stretching should never be painful, but it's normal to feel slightly uncomfortable while holding a stretch—a discomfort you might describe as "gentle tension." Once you feel this, you are benefiting from the stretch and don't have to move any further. Over time, as you become more flexible, you will be able to move further into the stretch before feeling this tension. You should choose stretches for each section of your body—upper, midsection, and lower. As was touched on earlier, it is a good idea to find a qualified fitness professional to help you set up a program appropriate for you.

Safety Tips for Stretching

- Warm up before you stretch. Muscles are like elastics. If you put an elastic in the freezer and then try to stretch it, it will likely break, but if you warm it up in the oven, it will stretch very easily. Muscles are the same. They need to be warmed up before they are stretched. This way there will be little chance of injury.
- Move into a stretch slowly and then hold it. Avoid any bouncing or jerky movements.
- Aim for a stretched, relaxed feeling without excessive tension or extreme discomfort.
- Breathe naturally; avoid holding your breath.

Conclusion

Exercise should be a lifelong commitment. This gives you plenty of time to make your program more challenging. Start yourself off slowly and very comfortably, with the idea of building up gradually as your fitness level improves. Get used to the activities you've chosen before you increase the level of difficulty. By doing what feels comfortable, you're giving your body the chance to let you know well in advance when you've had enough and it's time to stop. Keep in mind that exercise doesn't have to be pumping weights in the gym. By trying different types of activity, from team sports to partner walking, from fitness classes to stretching in your living room, you will find something that best suits you. Whenever questions arise, make sure you speak with your health-care provider. Happy exercising!

7

NUTRITION FOR OPTIMAL HEALTH

Dietary habits and food choices play a significant role in any anti-aging program. The old saying "You are what you eat" is ever so true. Wise dietary choices help you optimize your health, fight off chronic disease, and enhance your longevity. Advice offered by Hippocrates is worth remembering: "Let food be your medicine."

Components of Nutrition

The basic components of the human diet are referred to as *macronutrients*, namely protein, carbohydrates, fats, and water. To achieve optimal health, it is essential that you understand the roles of these macronutrients and maintain a proper balance of them in the food you eat.

Protein

Protein, which makes up 14 percent of your total weight, is necessary for building healthy bones, hair, nails, skin, and muscles. It provides you with energy and is needed in the manufacture of hormones, antibodies, and enzymes. In the body, the protein in food is broken down into amino acids, required for virtually every bodily function. The amino acids produced by the body are called *nonessential*, since they don't need to be obtained through diet. The *essential* amino acids must be provided by the food you eat.

Protein is found in both animal- and plant-based foods. Animal products like meat, poultry, eggs, cheese, and milk supply *complete proteins*, providing all the essential amino acids. Plant-based proteins found in such foods as beans, soy products, legumes, and nuts are called *incomplete proteins* because they lack some essential amino acids. However, if you choose your plants wisely and eat them in combination, you can obtain all the essential amino acids. For example, oats, lentils, and sunflower seeds eaten together or separately throughout the day provide all the essential amino acids. Plant proteins offer some health advantage, as they are often high in fiber and don't contain saturated fat. Soy protein, for example, lowers cholesterol and triglyceride levels significantly and offers protection against bone loss.[1]

Most health authorities recommend that you consume approximately 15–20 percent of total caloric intake from protein.[2] The recommended daily allowance for protein, based on body weight, is 0.8 grams per kilogram of body weight.[3] A higher intake is required for athletes, children, adolescents, and pregnant or lactating women. Be aware that eating too much protein can cause stress to the kidneys and a reduction in bone density.[4] Consult with a dietitian to determine your optimal protein intake.

Carbohydrates

Carbohydrates provide valuable nutrients and are sources of energy. There are two types of carbs, simple and complex. *Simple carbohydrates* include naturally occurring sugars (those in milk and fruit, for example) as well as the refined sugars (granulated sugar, corn syrup) that are added to foods. There's a big difference between these simple carbohydrates: fruits offer a range of nutrients and fiber, while refined sugars provide no nutritional value but a lot of calories and an increased risk of dental problems, high triglyceride levels, and low HDL (good) cholesterol.[5]

Complex carbohydrates are found in grains (wheat, rice, and oats), vegetables, and legumes. They provide vital nutrients such as the B vitamins, magnesium, zinc, selenium, vitamin E, and fiber. The health benefits of dietary fiber are numerous: it promotes bowel regularity (prevents constipation), regulates blood sugar, lowers cholesterol, reduces the risk of colon and breast cancer, and plays a role in weight management.[6] Unfortunately, many of us don't consume the recommended 25–35 grams per day of dietary fiber. You can increase your fiber intake by choosing whole, fresh, unrefined grains such as whole wheat bread, brown rice, and oatmeal. Raw or steamed vegetables and more beans and legumes in your diet will also help. Most authorities recommend that carbohydrates constitute about 55–65 percent of your total caloric intake.[7]

Another benefit of eating high-fiber complex carbohydrates is that they have a lower *glycemic index* (GI). The GI measures the impact of different foods on blood-sugar levels. The scale goes from 0 to 100, with 100 being the GI of pure glucose. Foods that are readily broken down and absorbed into the bloodstream cause a rapid increase in blood sugar and therefore have a higher GI. Foods that have a high GI include white bread, rice, sugar, honey, bananas, pineapple, apricots, potatoes, corn, and alcohol. The GI of these foods ranges from 70 to 100. In general, high-fiber foods have a lower GI. Whole grains, eggs, meats, and dairy products have a low GI. Foods classified as having a low GI have a rating of 50 or less.

Foods with a high glycemic index can cause a rapid increase in blood glucose and insulin levels, effects that can be hard on the pancreas and lead to mood swings, foggy head, and weakness. Since high insulin levels encourage the body to store more fat, foods with a high GI (even if they are carbohydrates) contribute to weight gain and obesity.

Fats

The Good News

As our main stored form of energy, fat is a major source of fuel. It is needed for proper growth and development, and it aids in the absorption of fat-soluble vitamins (A, D, E, and K). Yet many of us shy away from fat, when all we really need to do is distinguish between the good fats and the bad ones.

The good fats are the unsaturated fats, namely the monounsaturated and polyunsaturated fatty acids found in some vegetable oils (canola, olive, safflower), nuts, seeds, fish, beans, and some grains. These fats provide the essential fatty acids (EFAs) that are essential for good health. There are three EFAs: linoleic acid (LA, an omega-6 fatty acid), alpha-linoleic acid (LNA, an omega-3 fatty acid), and arachidonic acid (AA). All three are crucial in the development of the brain, inner ear, eyes, adrenal glands, and sex organs, and provide other health benefits as well. Diets rich in omega-3 fatty acids offer cardio-protection by lowering blood cholesterol and triglyceride levels, reducing blood clotting, and reducing the risk of heart attack and sudden death.[8] These fats aren't made in the body and so must be obtained through diet or supplementation.

Many reports suggest that the average diet doesn't provide enough EFAs and that we are getting too many omega-6 and not enough omega-3 EFAs. Virtually all age-related diseases have been linked to this improper balance (this issue will be discussed in further detail in Chapter 10).

Good food sources of LA and LNA include safflower seed oil, sunflower seed oil, sesame seed oil, hemp seed oil, flaxseed, and flaxseed oil. Some of the best sources of the omega-3 fatty acids are fish oils (salmon, mackerel, herring). The evidence for EFA is so convincing that the American Heart Association recommends increasing our intake of cold-water fish to at least two servings a week.[9]

Ground or milled flaxseed has a great nutty flavor and is an excellent addition to cereals and yogurt. Safflower or olive oil can be used in salad dressings. When cooking with oil, use olive or canola, since they are most resistant to damage by heating. Choose "unrefined" seed oils that are cold-pressed and sold in opaque (amber) glass bottles. Oils that provide a blend of LA and LNA in a proper ratio (Udo's Oil, for example) are among the most highly recommended EFA supplements on the market.

Fats to Avoid: Saturated Fats and Trans Fatty Acids

Saturated fats are found in animal products—meat, poultry, regular milk, cheese, butter, and lard, as well as in tropical oils (palm, palm kernel, coconut oil) and foods made from these oils. Many studies have linked diets high in saturated fat to heart disease, high cholesterol, obesity, and cancers of the breast, colon, and prostate.[10] The average North American adult gets 38 percent of the day's calories from fat, although health authorities suggest that no more than 30 percent should come from fat and less than 10 percent of that should be from saturated fat.[11]

Trans fatty acids occur naturally in small amounts in animal products and can be created when oils undergo a chemical process (hydrogenation) to make them solid at room temperature. Many margarines, for example, are hydrogenated. Trans fat is also found in cookies, crackers, and baked goods. The health risks of trans fatty acids include elevated cholesterol, heart disease, and heart attack.[12] Evidence also links them to cancer, particularly breast cancer.[13] Food companies have developed ways to make margarines without the hydrogenation and trans fat. Some new spreads even help lower cholesterol. Examples of healthy spreads are Promise and Becel™.

Cholesterol

Cholesterol, a waxy substance found in the fats (lipids) in our blood, is manufactured in the liver and also obtained from the diet. Our bodies need cholesterol to function properly; our sex hormones are produced from cholesterol, and it is essential for a healthy nervous system. Too much cholesterol, though, clogs arteries and increases the risk of heart disease.[14] A number of factors are known to elevate cholesterol levels: a diet high in saturated fat, cholesterol and trans fat, family history, lack of activity, and liver disorders.

Cholesterol is carried through the bloodstream by lipoproteins, namely, low-density lipoprotein (LDL) and high density lipoprotein (HDL). LDL is the main carrier and is often called "bad" cholesterol because it can build up in the artery walls and lead to atherosclerosis (a risk factor for heart attack and stroke).

Apo-lipoprotein (Lp_a) is a variation of LDL that is even more dangerous. Being very sticky, it adheres strongly to the artery walls and has recently been identified as a significant risk factor for heart disease.[15]

HDL cholesterol is refered to as "good" cholesterol because it picks up the LDL cholesterol deposited in the arteries and transports it to the liver to be broken down and eliminated. Most of us can lower our LDL levels by raising our HDL levels through moderate exercise and diet modification. Smoking has been shown to lower HDL.

Triglycerides (TG), another form of fat, are found in both animal and plant foods. They consist of a glycerol molecule and three fatty acids. TGs are measured in the blood and often checked with cholesterol levels. A diet high in fat, sugar, refined carbohydrates, and alcohol can elevate TGs. Overeating can also contribute, since excess carbohydrates and protein are converted to fat in the liver and then into TGs to be transported in the blood. High TG levels are associated with chronic disease, particularly heart disease and diabetes, and can occur even if blood cholesterol is normal; it's thus important to get TG levels checked regularly. In most cases, these levels can be effectively managed with diet and exercise.

Water

Though often taken for granted, pure water is essential to our health. Our bodies, after all, are approximately 70 percent water. Water helps our bodies perform many important functions, including the transport of nutrients, body temperature regulation, and the removal of waste. A minimum of 8–10 glasses daily is generally recommended, more if you exercise vigorously.

Guidelines for Healthy Eating

You can eat well by monitoring the quality, variety, and quantity of your food. Nutrient-rich foods, functional foods, and a reduced caloric intake can help you achieve a healthier and longer life. If necessary, supplements can fill in any nutritional gaps you may have, ensuring a complete diet.

The Importance of Quality

Focus on fresh raw fruits and vegetables, looking for color and variety. These foods should constitute most of your caloric intake. Try to buy organic produce as often as possible. Minimize the storage time and the cooking and reheating of produce; nutrient value diminishes with time and overcooking.

Choose whole grains (brown rice, oats, multi-grain breads) over the refined and processed varieties. Refined grains, like white flour, have had most of their vitamins and minerals removed. Minimize sugar intake (use pureed fruit, honey, or stevia instead), and eliminate food additives and preservatives where possible.

Functional Foods

According to the International Food Information Council, functional foods are "foods that offer health benefits beyond basic nutrition." Specifically, they have value in the prevention and treatment of disease. Here are some examples of functional foods and their associated health claims:[16]

Oat bran   Oat bran contains a soluble fiber called beta-glucan that lowers cholesterol. Regular consumption of oat bran has been associated with a reduced incidence of coronary heart disease.

Green tea Green tea is rich in polyphenols, which neutralize free radicals and reduce the risk of cancer. Black tea offers similar benefits.

Garlic Clinical studies have shown that garlic reduces cholesterol and suppresses the harmful effects of LDL cholesterol oxidation (the process whereby LDL cholesterol chemically changes and adheres to the vessel wall—the beginning of atherosclerosis). Preliminary evidence suggests that garlic has some antithrombotic activity (reducing blood clotting). A diet generous in garlic has also been linked to decreased risks of laryngeal, gastric, and endometrial cancers and colorectal polyps.[17] Those of you who don't like the taste or smell of garlic can get the benefits of garlic in supplement form. The most widely studied garlic supplement on the market is Kyolic™ aged garlic extract. (See Appendix 7.1.)

Soybeans Soybeans contain isoflavones, which help reduce cholesterol, fight cancer, increase bone density, and reduce menopausal symptoms. In 1999 the U.S. Food and Drug Administration acknowledged the heart-health benefits of soy on the basis of clinical studies showing that it reduces total and LDL cholesterol. Scientific studies show that 25 grams of soy protein daily is needed to produce a significant cholesterol-lowering effect. Aside from in tofu, you can get soy protein in soy nuts, yogurts, bars, or shakes.

Flaxseed The lignans in flaxseed offer protection against heart disease by lowering LDL cholesterol, total cholesterol, and triglyceride levels, and may also reduce cancer risk.

Broccoli The sulphoraphane in broccoli neutralizes free radicals and may reduce the risk of cancer. Sulphoraphane is also found in kale and horseradish.

Yogurt Yogurt contains active bacteria cultures that promote a healthy intestinal tract. These cultures also help you digest the naturally occurring sugar (lactose) in dairy products that causes bloating and diarrhea in some people. Yogurt also contains protein, calcium, magnesium, riboflavin, vitamins B6 and B12, and more. Avoid the "diet" or "light" yogurts, since they are sweetened with aspartame, a chemical whose safety in food is questionable.

The Importance of Variety

To ensure that you get a broad range of nutrients in your diet, rotate your food choices. That way, you won't be eating the same foods all the time. If you choose from a narrow selection, however, you might miss out on some very important vitamins and minerals. A varied diet, rich in plant foods, will maximize your nutrient intake. Experiment with new foods and recipes, and retry those previously disliked foods.

The Importance of Quantity

Eat small, frequent meals at regular intervals, and try not to vary the times of daily meals. This helps to prevent imbalances in metabolism and fluctuations in blood-sugar levels; it also reduces the risk of overeating. You shouldn't skip meals, even if you're trying to lose weight, since this can cause your body to enter starvation mode and retain fat. Control portions. For example, a serving equals one piece of fruit, one cup of raw or half a cup of cooked vegetables, one slice of bread, half a cup of cooked rice or pasta, or 2–3 ounces of meat. Eat slowly and chew your food thoroughly. A meal should last 20–30 minutes.

Caloric Restriction Optimal Nutrition (CRON)

There is another reason to control portions—you will live longer! Caloric restriction leads to weight loss, which can improve health parameters in overweight individuals but also benefits the non-obese. A recent study involving monkeys showed that a 30 percent caloric restriction can lead to a 25-point elevation in HDL (good) cholesterol, a 20-point decrease in triglycerides, and a small but significant decrease in blood pressure.[18] Interestingly, the monkeys were not obese. This research was significant in that it showed health benefits and increased longevity with caloric restriction in lean animals. Other studies have linked caloric restriction to better glucose tolerance and insulin sensitivity, improved blood-sugar levels, and reduced insulin secretion (lowering the risk of Type 2 diabetes).

Another study found that a 30 percent reduction in calories slowed the decline of the hormone DHEA (dehydroepiandrosterone),[19] a naturally occurring hormone in the body that declines with age, therefore acting as an important marker of the rate of aging. While DHEA supplements are often promoted as "the fountain of youth," studies have not proven that they offer benefits to longevity. It is thought that it is more important to slow the natural decline in DHEA than to increase levels with supplements later in life.

In Okinawa, Japan, there are more than four times the number of centenarians than elsewhere in Japan and certainly more than in North America. How do the Okinawans' diets differ? They eat three times more vegetables, two times more fish, and consume one-third fewer calories. Recent research has indeed shown that people who follow a low-calorie, nutrient-rich diet can extend their life span, reduce brain aging, and lower the risk of degenerative disease.[20]

As you restrict calories, the effort needed by your body to digest food also decreases, reducing the production of free radicals and oxidative stress. Fewer free radicals mean less cellular damage and less wear and tear on organ systems. This improves your body's ability to deal with metabolic by-products and allows your organ systems to function optimally. The result is an extended life span.

Caloric restriction also leads to a sharper mind and clearer thinking by stimulating the release of chemicals that protect brain cells. Evidence suggests that the brain's capacity for self-repair can be enhanced through dietary modifications.

Caloric restriction means limiting calories to the amount needed for optimal functioning of the body. It is not intended to cause starvation or malnutrition; nutritional deficiencies can accelerate aging. A low-calorie diet would include about 1,800 calories per day, far less than what the average North American consumes. Your goal is to exercise portion control and choose nutrient-dense foods.

Nutritional Supplements

Despite your best intentions, it can be difficult to get all the required nutrients from diet alone. Moreover, there are circumstances that increase the need for vitamins and minerals—pregnancy, exposure to stress, smoking, and exposure to environmental toxins, to name a few. Mounting research has demonstrated the benefits of nutritional supplements in optimizing health and in treating and preventing disease. At a minimum, a good-quality multivitamin and mineral supplement should be considered. A green food supplement like greens+™ is another wise choice, especially for those unable to eat the recommended 5–10 servings of fruit and vegetables per day. One serving of greens+™ is equivalent to six servings of vegetables, providing a good source of fiber, vitamins, minerals, and plant-based (phyto-) nutrients.

Food Allergies and Intolerances

Most people will enjoy better health by following the above dietary guidelines, but certain individuals may have problems with certain foods. While food allergies or food intolerances affect nearly everyone at some point,[21] in many cases they go undetected because the symptoms can be subtle or difficult to diagnose.

Food allergies occur when the immune system overreacts to proteins in certain foods. More than 200 food ingredients can evoke allergic reactions. Among the most common food allergies are nuts, milk, eggs, shellfish, and wheat. Symptoms may include skin rash, hives, sinus congestion, wheezing, nausea, and headache. In extreme cases, an anaphylactic reaction can be life threatening, causing swelling of the tongue and throat and a sharp decline in blood pressure.

Food intolerances are not true allergies; rather they involve the body's inability to digest certain components of food. The reactions are often less severe than allergic reactions. They include headache, nausea, constipation, diarrhea, fatigue, eczema, rash, and muscle aches. The most common food intolerances occur with gluten (celiac disease), sulfites, lactose, monosodium glutamate (MSG), food colors, and chocolate.

The Elimination Diet

The Elimination Diet was developed by HealthComm International Inc. as a strategy to determine and ultimately remove from the diet allergens that could be hindering digestion and causing food allergies or intolerances. In clinical practice, this diet has been found to help regulate blood sugar, reduce cholesterol and blood pressure, control body weight, and improve energy levels, mood, and sleep quality.

Guidelines for the Modified Elimination Diet are given in Appendix 7. This appendix also includes a list of recommended foods and foods to avoid. For best results, follow the diet carefully for at least one month. Although it is strict, its health benefits make it worthwhile. This diet does not restrict calories and will not make you feel hungry. The main point is to prepare meals from the foods allowed. After the diet is followed for one month, you can gradually reintroduce foods one at a time in weekly intervals. Start by adding beef, then eggs, then gluten-containing grains other than wheat, then wheat, and lastly dairy. For example, have one serving of beef during the first week. Pay close attention to how you feel. Wait one week before you reintroduce the next food. If you notice any adverse health effects from a reintroduced food, you can conclude that this is a food to avoid.

Depending on your health status, a variety of medical food products may be recommended as supplements to the Elimination Diet. Consult your doctor about using UltraBalance™ medical foods along with the diet.

Fasting

In Chapter 2 we discussed various theories of aging, including the Wear and Tear Theory. According to this theory, aging is accelerated by the overload of toxins in our environment, food, water, air, drugs, and other factors. As the body loses its ability to renew and rid itself of these toxins, damage and decay occur. Even without these external forces, the body produces toxins through normal metabolic processes. Fasting is one method of eliminating toxins from the body. Its health benefits include improved elimination, reduced toxic buildup, improved immune function and tissue repair, reduced pain and inflammation, clearer skin, weight reduction, and better concentration.

It is very important to consult a health-care practitioner before initiating a fast.

Conclusion

In this chapter, we learned that food can be used as a tool to ward off disease and extend our life span. The optimal anti-aging diet focuses on a variety of quality foods that are low in calories but high in nutrients. Fresh raw vegetables and fruits, whole grains, and lean protein sources should be your mainstays. Make changes gradually and think of this as a healthy way of eating rather than as a diet. Eating healthy food can be both fun and rewarding.

PART 3

STRATEGIES, PROTOCOLS, AND THERAPIES

8

THE ROLE OF HORMONES

If you are looking for the fountain of youth, sorry, it doesn't exist and it likely never will. This truth, though, hasn't stopped the promulgation of hormone replacement therapy (HRT) as an elixir for long life. Today's popular anti-aging equation seems to be that old age can be beaten if you just restore the levels of major hormones to those seen in youth. Yes, most hormones decline as people age, but as noted earlier, hormonal fluctuations are not causes of aging or age-related disease—they're merely the observed effects or symptoms of aging.

Aging is chronic, and any chronic biological process—whether diseased or not—has many causes. Thus, if you want to modify the way you'll age, you need to address the root causes of diseased aging. You can't simply treat the effects or symptoms of aging and expect long-lasting results.

The goal of this chapter is to help you improve hormone balance so as to optimize metabolism. You will learn more about the negative effects of excessive cortisol and insulin, the importance of stable blood-sugar levels, and the effects of poor thyroid function. We begin by looking at the two hormones most critical in the pursuit of extended youth: cortisol and insulin.

What Is Cortisol?

While virtually all hormones decline or are maintained in the aging process, the stress hormone cortisol increases. Faced with any type of stress (mental, emotional, physical, environmental), the body responds by producing cortisol. Cortisol mobilizes stored reserves of sugar, fat, protein, vitamins, and minerals and sends them into the bloodstream to the parts of the body that need them most to cope with the ordeal of stress. If stress is extreme, especially if every situation is perceived as threatening, cortisol levels rise.

DIAGRAM 8.1: Main Hormones Produced from Cholesterol

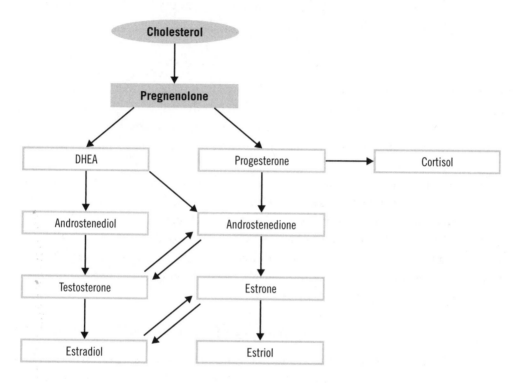

Pregnenolone is the major hormone produced from cholesterol. Pregnenolone can go on to produce testosterone, the three major estrogens (estrone, estradiol, and estriol), and progesterone. As the need for cortisol increases (as required to meet the demands of chronic stress during the aging process), the production of these aforementioned hormones declines more rapidly.

The Effects of Cortisol on Liver Function

The adrenal glands produce cortisol from cholesterol. Now, the liver produces about 80 percent of the cholesterol floating around in your blood; dietary sources account for the rest, about 20 percent. As Diagram 8.1 makes clear, cholesterol plays an extremely important role in the body. All steroidal hormones, in fact, are derived from this misunderstood fat molecule. When you're constantly under stress, most of your cholesterol is converted to cortisol and the production of all other hormones declines, a process that occurs more rapidly during the aging process. When there's a high demand for cortisol, the liver tries to keep up by producing and storing more cholesterol, causing blood cholesterol levels to rise. Of course, you help out by ingesting fatty foods (people under severe stress crave fatty foods). At some point the liver becomes infiltrated with fat and struggles to detoxify the body. The waste and toxins that accumulate in the blood are eventually deposited in your tissues and fat stores. This puts a tremendous load on the lymphatic system, whose function is to remove waste for excretion.

The Effects of Cortisol on Immune Function

Too much stress-derived cortisol causes the lymphatic system to shrink and become congested. The lymphatic system is a highway along which waste is carried from your tissues and through which white blood cells travel to get to sites of injury and infection. Thus, with poor lymphatic flow, not only are toxins and wastes not readily cleared, but overall immune function is affected.

Swollen and sore lymph nodes and poor skin health and color are among the symptoms of a clogged lymphatic system. Others are chronic sore throats and congested mucous membranes (sinuses, lungs, gastrointestinal tract, urinary tract). Also, with poor lymphatic drainage, allergies develop. Moreover, because the body cannot readily eliminate toxins with a faulty lymphatic system, it tends to retain water. Swollen face, legs, and ankles at the end of the day, as well as pressure headaches and feelings of heaviness and fatigue, are other signs of a sluggish lymphatic system.

The Effects of Cortisol on Brain Function

Even your brain and nervous system are not spared from the ever-pervasive effects of excessive cortisol. Under the mercy of cortisol, your coping mechanisms falter. You become easily angered and frustrated, and your concentration and memory begin to fail. Depression in all its forms becomes very likely. Chronically elevated amounts of cortisol literally destroy various regions of the brain. Here are just some of the major problems created when your system sees ocean waves of cortisol:

- Cognitive impairment (short-term memory loss, poor concentration and focus)
- Depression
- Elevated blood glucose
- Elevated blood cholesterol
- Elevated blood pressure (water and sodium retention)
- Fatigue
- Fatty liver and impaired detoxification
- Impaired digestion and elimination

- Increased excretion of nutrients (calcium, magnesium, potassium, vitamin C, and the B vitamins)
- Insomnia
- Loss of sexual desire
- Menstrual-cycle disturbances
- Osteoporosis
- Suppressed thyroid function
- Weight gain (central obesity)
- Weakened immune function

The questionnaire in Appendix 8.1 will help you determine your own cortisol level.

The Effects on the Adrenal Glands of Excessive Cortisol Demand

Your adrenal glands, which produce cortisol, get larger in size to meet the high demand for this stress hormone. However, at some point, and it's only a matter of time and the level of stress in your life, the adrenal glands shrink in size and become exhausted. When adrenal exhaustion sets in, you become physically and mentally fatigued. Dark circles develop under your eyes, and generally you look worn out. You have trouble getting a good night's sleep and struggle to get up in the morning. You crave sweet and/or salty fatty foods when your adrenals are tired, and you become achier and may get frequent headaches. Chronic conditions like asthma or migraines become worse, since your adrenal glands are responsible for controlling all types of inflammatory disorders. When your adrenals are exhausted, all of life's challenges seem enormous—everything overwhelms you.

What Is Insulin Resistance?

When you swim in the river of stress, some degree of insulin resistance develops. Recall that cortisol raises the level of sugar in the blood in order to make it available to the cells of the body that need it; the pancreas, meanwhile, secretes insulin to deliver the sugar to these cells. However, with constant increases in blood sugar (caused by excessive cortisol), the body produces even more insulin. With prolonged elevated levels of insulin, your cells will at some point fail to respond properly; we call this phenomenon *insulin resistance* (see Chapters 2 and 3). The equation is simple: more cortisol, more sugar, and more insulin = insulin resistance.

Just as cortisol tends to rise during the aging process, so too does insulin. No one can afford to incur insulin resistance as a debit if they hope to maximize their functional life span. As mentioned in Chapters 2 and 3, insulin resistance can lead to a range of diseases and conditions, the most common being age-related fatigue. Here's a list of the major complications resulting from insulin resistance:

- Allergies
- Autoimmune diseases
- Cognitive impairment
- Chronic inflammatory disorders
- Diabetes (Type 2)
- Endometriosis
- Fibroids
- Fatigue
- Hardening and narrowing of arteries/poor circulation
- High cholesterol
- High uric acids
- Hormonal disturbances (PMS, menopausal, etc.)
- Hypertension
- Hypothyroidism
- Impaired detoxification
- Obesity
- Polycystic ovary syndrome

Typically, as insulin levels rise during the aging process and some degree of insulin resistance is established, the body has great difficulty regulating blood sugar. *Dysglycemia* is a condition where there are huge fluctuations in blood sugar, going from high (hyperglycemia) to low (hypoglycemia) and vice versa. Missing breakfast or going for more than six to eight hours without eating makes it hard for your system to maintain your blood-sugar level. When blood sugar spikes and plummets, you function like a yo-yo, up one minute and down the next.

Whether or not you have diabetes, you should take note of the following signs and symptoms of dysglycemia:

- Anxiety
- Blurred vision
- Depression
- Emotional difficulties, fearfulness, irritability, and mood swings
- Heart palpitations
- Headache, dizziness, light-headedness
- Constant hunger, craving sugary sweets
- Hyperactivity, jitteriness, nervousness
- Inability to focus or concentrate
- Insomnia, disturbing dreams
- Indecisiveness
- Labored breathing
- Mental and physical fatigue

- Stomach nervousness
- Sweating, spontaneous or excessive

The Effects of Poor Thyroid Function

Prolonged surges of cortisol can eventually suppress the function of the thyroid gland. *Hypothyroidism* (an underactive thyroid), a common phenomenon as people get older, is an indication of the effects of stress-induced cortisol. Hypothyroidism tends to affect more women than men of advancing years. The thyroid gland is not only responsible for physical and mental well-being; it also helps control weight, body temperature, and overall metabolism. See the following signs and symptoms of a sub-par thyroid gland. If you suffer from many of these, you may require supervised medical treatment.

- Anemia
- Anxiety, agitation
- Constipation
- Decreased sexual drive (both men and women)
- Depression
- Fatigue
- Dry, coarse, thinning, or falling-out hair
- Headache
- High cholesterol
- Inability to tolerate cold temperatures; cold hands and feet
- Insomnia
- Infertility (both men and women)
- Menstrual irregularities
- Muscular weakness and/or pain
- Weak, brittle, or ridged nails
- Poor memory and mental focus; confusion and dullness
- Tingling in fingers
- Skin changes (dry, pale, cool)
- Wounds slow to heal; prolonged recovery from infections
- Slow heart rate
- Slow and/or slurred speech, hoarseness
- Water retention (mainly hands and feet)
- Weight gain and inability to lose weight

Improving Stress Response with Adaptogens

The key to controlling the hormonal mess seen in aging is to deal better with stress. Fortunately, there is a class of medicines known as *adaptogens* that can help. Adaptogens are natural, plant-based products that have been shown to protect the body when it is under stress. Specifically, adaptogens improve all three phases of stress identified by Dr. Hans Selye: alarm, resistance, and exhaustion (see Chapter 5). A number of adaptogens have been shown to increase the body's capacity to deal with and recover from stress.

The product Panax Ginseng C.A. Meyer (commercially available as Ginsana; see Appendix 7.1) is an adaptogen that under various stress-induced situations improves physical and mental performance, immune function, and maintenance of adrenal gland size and function. Like all adaptogens, Panax Ginseng can restore the body's systems and chemicals to their proper balance regardless of what, specifically, has been affected. For instance, ginseng will raise cortisol levels of non-diabetic individuals so that they can deal with stress more efficiently. Conversely, ginseng will lower cortisol levels in diabetic individuals, reducing the need for insulin and allowing for better sugar regulation. Thus, ginseng's effects are quite variable on blood-sugar levels, lowering or raising it depending on the need.[1] Appendix 8.2 contains a list of adaptogens (more formally called *adaptogenic phytomedicines*) and the variety of observed effects.

Some adaptogens are better at supporting specific functions than others. Astragalus, a great immunity booster, helps those susceptible to infection when under stress, while American ginseng has "cooling" properties that make it useful for people who are emotionally volatile under stress. Rhodiola is ideal for individuals who are mentally troubled and experience heart palpitations when under stress. Some products combine several adaptogens and have a broad-spectrum action.[2] If you choose to go this route, it's best to have a health-care professional help you decide on the appropriate adaptogen(s), dose, and length of treatment. If you are taking prescription medicines, first seek clearance from your doctor.

Improving Stress Response with Supplements

The Great Conqueror: Vitamin C

Commercially available since the late 1930s, vitamin C is the most widely taken vitamin supplement. Vitamin C greatly aids the adrenal glands in dealing with the stress response. It also helps in the production of important neurotransmitters that are required for good mood and proper sleep. Prolonged or poorly handled stress, chronic disease, and the stress of aging itself drastically reduce the levels of vitamin C. If your body becomes depleted of vitamin C, you tend to have difficulty handling added stress. Here is a list of the many roles played by vitamin C in ensuring healthy aging:[3]

Cardiovascular Support

- Aids in the metabolism and elimination of cholesterol and thus keeps blood cholesterol levels in check
- Prevents LDL cholesterol from oxidizing and sticking to arteries and thereby clogging circulation
- Strengthens the integrity of blood vessels and thus helps maintain optimal circulation
- Keeps blood vessels well dilated, thereby preventing high blood pressure and helping to lower it if it is high

Immune Support

- Increases the number of immune system cells and improves their function of fighting infection of all kinds
- Prevents the body from developing allergies and helps it deal with existing allergies
- Helps to heal skin wounds, other damaged tissues, and organs
- Helps to prevent cancer from spreading

Connective Tissue Support

- Is needed in the production of collagen and thus is essential for healthy skin, gums, teeth, bones, ligaments, tendons, cartilage, and the discs of the vertebrae

Antioxidant Support

- Helps to neutralize free radicals and repair the damage they do
- Increases the production of other compounds needed to neutralize free radicals

Metabolic Support

- Helps to regulate blood sugar and protect the body from the damaging effects of elevated sugar levels
- Helps the thyroid gland produce thyroid hormones that, among many things, are needed to control weight and energy levels, maintain good mood, and ensure proper sleep
- Helps in the production of carnitine, an amino acid that helps burn fat, thereby controlling weight gain

You need to eat at least five servings of fresh fruits and vegetables daily to meet the minimum required amounts of vitamin C. Since it is difficult to get optimal amounts from diet alone, we recommend that most adults take 500–1,000 milligrams of vitamin C on a daily basis. If you feel swamped by stress, are susceptible to infection, or have a chronic degenerative disease, you might find doses higher than 1,000 milligrams daily to be quite helpful. While vitamin C supplementation is extremely safe, ideally you should seek professional advice about the optimal dose for you.

The Buzz of B Vitamins

Stress of any kind depletes your body of all the B vitamins. Depletion takes place at different rates in different people. You quite likely have heard that the B vitamins should be taken as a complex supplement to better deal with stress. While this is true, we would like to highlight some members of the vitamin B family that may be needed in higher amounts.[4]

Vitamin B1 or thiamin   This vitamin is critical in metabolizing glucose to be converted for energy. It helps in the production of acetylcholine, an important neurotransmitter used for optimal nerve and brain function. Sufficient levels of vitamin B1 are needed for memory and maintaining good mood in times of stress and illness. It is commonly known as the morale vitamin.

Vitamin B2   Niacin and the derivative niacinamide are this vitamin's two major forms. It helps insulin work better, thereby stabilizing blood sugar; it also helps the adrenal glands produce estrogen, progesterone, testosterone, and other important hormones depleted through stress. Sufficient levels of niacinamide are needed to promote calmness.

Vitamin B5 or pantothenic acid   Vitamin B5 helps maintain optimal adrenal gland function and prevent or delay stress-induced fatigue. It also helps prevent low blood sugar. It is commonly known as the anti-stress vitamin because it helps the body adapt to stress.

Vitamin B6 or pyridoxine   Vitamin B6 helps with the production and function of all hormones and neurotransmitters and thereby ensures balance in stressful situations. It also helps regulate blood-sugar levels, helps the body use protein as a fuel source more efficiently, helps remove waste and excessive water, and helps build healthy nerve tissue.

Blood-Sugar Supplements

All the detrimental changes seen in aging and age-related disease can be treated and perhaps even avoided with better blood-sugar control. Remember, high levels of cortisol block the action of insulin, making blood sugar erratic. Thus, coping better with the cause of high cortisol levels—stress—is critical. The following are some of the nutrients that can be helpful in improving insulin sensitivity and controlling blood sugar.

Chromium   By improving insulin's efficiency, chromium lowers elevated blood-sugar levels and the need for more insulin. It also lowers cholesterol and triglycerides, and during exercise, can burn fat and increase muscle mass.

Zinc   This mineral is required for the production, secretion, and utilization of insulin. It protects insulin from free-radical damage, thus enabling insulin to perform its function in regulating blood sugar.

Vitamin E   This vitamin's antioxidant properties protect cells and allow insulin to better bind onto the body's cells in regulating blood sugar. The best supplemental form of this vitamin includes the entire family of vitamin E compounds (referred to as the tocopherols); it is commercially available as "mixed E."

Magnesium   This mineral is the best friend of your nerves, muscles, and heart, as it prevents these tissues from being overstimulated under stress. Sufficient levels are needed to keep you relaxed and focused and to ensure adequate sleep. Commonly known as the anti-stress mineral, it helps to stabilize blood sugar.

Alpha lipoic acid   The best form of this vitamin, known as (R+) lipoic acid, has unique broad-spectrum antioxidant properties. It sensitizes cells to insulin and thereby helps in blood-sugar regulation.

Essential fatty acids   Omega-6 fatty acids are found in evening primrose oil; omega-3 fatty acids are found in flaxseed oil and fish oil. Both types are needed to allow insulin to better bind to cells.

Thyroid Supplements

If you suspect that your thyroid is underactive, it is essential that you get the necessary blood tests through your doctor. Whether or not you have hypothyroidism and require medication, the following supplements can be useful. To get a good idea of how well your thyroid is regulating your overall metabolism, measure your basal body temperature; see Appendix 8.3 for details. The following are some recommended thyroid supplements:

Iodine   The thyroid gland needs this mineral for the production of thyroid hormones.

Selenium   This mineral activates thyroid hormones once they're in the bloodstream.

Vitamins A and D   These fat-soluble vitamins help the activated thyroid hormones bind to cells so that they can carry out their proper action.

Pulling It All Together

We started this chapter by discussing the far-reaching effects of excessive cortisol and insulin during the aging process. It's important to realize that keeping blood sugar steady helps you deal better with stress and lowers the levels of cortisol and insulin your body will see. When stress is prolonged and excessive, all other hormones decline. Unfortunately, just taking supplements for these declining hormones isn't the answer. Unless your cortisol, insulin, and blood sugar are well regulated, you can't expect to benefit from any type of hormone replacement. That's why, for women, estrogen replacement is not always a guarantee against hot flashes, heart disease, or bone loss. Furthermore, adding supplementary hormones to the biochemical mayhem described in this chapter increases the risk of cancer. Therefore, before buying into any hormone supplement's promise of youth and disease-free longevity, follow the basic program presented next.

The Basic Program

1. Evaluate your diet and make the necessary changes. Don't rely too much on one food group or source. Make sure you have moderation, variety, and balance in your diet. Know the signs and symptoms of irregular blood sugar. Balance your blood sugar by not skipping meals and bingeing with food. (See Chapter 7.)

2. Develop and follow an exercise program. (See Chapter 6.)

3. Identify and evaluate the stress in your life. Understand the positive and negative aspects of the effects of stress. Even though you may be "handling" stress just fine, the sheer amount of it and the lack of balance in your life will have inevitable health consequences. (See Chapters 3 and 5.)

4. Choose a high-quality multivitamin and mineral supplement to be taken three times a day with meals. This ensures a steady level of nutrients in your system throughout the day. There are many high-quality formulas available, for example, MULTI-FORCE™, manufactured by Prairie Naturals, is one that is based on extensive research. This specialized supplement provides the suggested optimum nutrient allowance (SONA) of multiple vitamins, minerals, and other health-promoting factors. The SONA includes significantly greater amounts of the nutrients required for optimum health than the RDA (recommended daily allowance), which only ensures prevention of nutrient-deficiency diseases. The levels of the SONA are based on a research study carried out by Dr. Emanuel Cheraskin and Dr. W.M. Ringsdorf at the University of Alabama Medical School in which 13,500 people were followed over a 15-year period.[5] Take one (or two, for intense use) easy-to-swallow capsules of MULTI-FORCE™ three times daily with meals. This supplement is available in powder form and can be mixed with juice for those who have difficulty swallowing. (See Appendix 6.) Unless there is an identified

need, avoid multivitamin supplements that contain iron, since iron can be problematic for men and women over 50.

5. Take through the course of the day 500–1,000 milligrams (or more if needed) of vitamin C. Multiple vitamin supplements rarely include amounts this large, so you generally need this additional supplement.

6. Take 400–800 IU of vitamin E daily (in a natural form that provides a mixture of all the compounds in the vitamin E family) on top of a high-quality multiple vitamin and mineral supplement. Vitamin E is better absorbed when taken with meals.

7. If you need help coping with stress, consider taking adaptogens. Be patient: it usually takes two to four weeks before beneficial effects of adaptogens are noticed. Take these supplements continuously for twelve weeks and then take a two-week break. Repeat the cycle, each time noting improvements so that you can judge whether you should be taking adaptogens on an ongoing basis in this fashion.

Conclusion

Since elevated levels of cortisol and insulin are universal age-related phenomena, everyone seeking healthy aging should try to keep these hormones in balance. The rate of decline and subsequent efficiency of every other hormone in the body hinge upon the balance of these two. No one can expect to benefit from any type of hormone therapy, natural or otherwise, until cortisol, insulin, and blood sugar are well regulated.

Don't circumvent what has been outlined in this chapter by rushing out and buying supplements. Remember this important health equation: poor lifestyle + poor diet + supplements = poor health.

Before reading further, you might want to review the earlier chapters—just to strengthen your foundation for better health and longevity. Then turn to the discussion of the digestive tract in Chapter 9. As you will see, a healthy digestive system lies at the root of good health. All other systems in the body depend on it.

9

DIGESTION: THE FAST TRACK TO GOOD HEALTH

In this chapter, we will look at why optimal digestion is important in ensuring healthy aging. You will become familiar with the various parts of the digestive tract, learn to identify the signs and symptoms of poor digestion, and find out what can be done to aid this process. Treatment options for chronic conditions and diseases of the digestive tract will also be discussed. Most importantly, you will learn why everyone should consider a cleansing and detoxification program.

The Digestive Process: The Origins of Good Health

During a person's lifetime, more than 30 tons of food pass through the digestive tract. When the gut (the small and large intestines) falters, rapid and diseased aging ensues. The origins of almost all chronic inflammatory disorders, including diseased aging, can be traced back to defects in the gut. Good health can only take root in good digestion. Your drive and passion for life depend on the intensity of your "intestinal fire."

The digestive process has three phases: breaking down food, absorbing nutrients, and eliminating waste.

Breaking Down Food

Digestion begins in the mouth. Chewing your food completely helps in three important ways. First, mechanically breaking down food into the smallest pieces possible puts less of a demand on the rest of the digestive system. Second, thoroughly chewing food ensures that the salivary glands secrete ample amounts of the enzymes needed to break down carbohydrate-rich foods. Last, patiently chewing food alerts the rest of the digestive system to get into gear.

The stomach is next in line. The hydrochloric acid (HCL) secreted in the stomach breaks down protein-rich foods and facilitates the absorption of many vitamins and minerals—calcium, magnesium, zinc, iron, beta carotene, and vitamins B and C. HCL also destroys harmful micro-organisms before they damage the gut and encourages the pancreas, liver, and gallbladder to perform their jobs to the fullest. During the aging process, there is generally a steady and significant decline in HCL secretion. Table 9.1 outlines problems associated with low HCL output.[1]

TABLE 9.1: Signs and Symptoms of Low HCL Output and Some Associated Diseases

Symptoms	Bloating, belching, burning, flatulence, fullness or heaviness shortly after meals
	Constipation or diarrhea
	Fatigue
	Multiple food intolerances and sensitivities
	Nausea shortly after taking supplements
	Rectal itching
Signs	Abnormal flora
	Chronic intestinal infections (bacterial, fungal, parasitic)
	Dilated blood vessels in cheeks and nose
	Hair loss
	Iron deficiency
	Weak, peeling, and cracked fingernails
	Undigested food in stool
Conditions and Diseases	Adult-onset acne or rosacea
	Autoimmune diseases
	Anemia
	Asthma
	Celiac disease
	Chronic hives
	Depression
	Diabetes
	Eczema
	Hypothyroidism
	Osteoporosis
	Psoriasis
	Ulcerative colitis

The Pancreas, Liver, and Gallbladder

Once food leaves the stomach, the pancreas and liver are almost simultaneously called upon to perform their digestive duties. The pancreas secretes enzymes (protease, amylase, and lipase) to break down protein, carbohydrates, and fats. It also secretes bicarbonate salts to neutralize the acid content of food that has left the stomach. Daily, as a result of eating, a total of two liters of pancreatic secretions are received in the intestines. Habitual overeating or eating in a tense and quick manner will eventually exhaust the pancreas.

When the pancreas begins to "dry up" during the aging process, certain problems arise. First, protein malabsorption occurs, making it difficult for the body to maintain muscle mass and repair connective tissue. Second, when insufficient protease is secreted, food (mainly protein and fat) is left in the intestine to rot. Harmful micro-organisms (bacteria, fungi, parasites) are given the opportunity to ferment this undigested food (a process known as putrefaction), producing toxins that damage the lining of the gut. Food allergies and intolerances are other consequences of the pancreas's inability to secrete enough enzymes.

As a digestive participant, the liver manufactures bile from cholesterol and secretes it via the gallbladder (where it is concentrated) into the small intestine. Bile has two basic functions. First, it ensures optimal absorption of dietary cholesterol, essential fatty acids, and fat-soluble vitamins (A, D, E, K). Second, it is via the bile that metabolic waste products are eliminated. Dietary fiber binds toxin-laden bile and literally pulls it out of the body; this keeps bile from stagnating in the gallbladder and prevents gallstone formation. When bile has performed its tasks and is removed, the liver can again make use of the cholesterol in the blood by producing more bile. This is how adequate fiber consumption keeps blood cholesterol levels in check.

The liver performs well over 500 different functions. Here is a list of the top 10:

1. Aids in digestion

2. Cleanses blood of metabolic waste and toxins

3. Regulates blood sugar

4. Helps the body burn fat and cholesterol

5. Supports immune function by destroying germs

6. Balances hormones

7. Stores iron and other vitamins and minerals in order to produce healthy red blood cells

8. Maintains healthy eyes, skin, hair, nails, and other connective tissue

9. Regulates the nervous system, ensuring good mood, optimal brain function, and proper sleep

10. Regulates blood viscosity, inflammation, and tissue repair

As you can see, your vitality and overall wellness depend on the health of your liver. Everyone, diseased or not, benefits from therapies designed to enhance liver function. Later on we will discuss what you can do to support your liver, but now we'll move to the second phase of digestion.

Absorption of Food

The lining of the small intestine secretes enzymes that help select the nutrients, such as vitamins and minerals, that are to be sent into the bloodstream. The small intestine also harbors beneficial bacteria that further break down food so that it can be fully assimilated. These friendly bacteria support the body in other ways as well: they reduce food allergies and intolerances; they produce vitamins B and K to be used by the body and to help process cholesterol; they protect the lining of the gut by destroying harmful bacteria, fungi, and parasites; and they regulate elimination, thereby preventing either diarrhea or constipation.[2] The small intestine acts as a barrier, keeping harmful micro-organisms, toxins, and food particles from entering the bloodstream. Its effectiveness as a barrier is directly dependent on its bacterial flora.

Up to 400 different species of bacteria line the gastrointestinal tract (the stomach and intestines), and their numbers are in the trillions. The balance in this microbial community determines overall health: for good health, the beneficial bacteria must outnumber their harmful counterparts.

Aging and stress lead to a reduction of the beneficial bacteria in the colon. This reduction allows the formation of toxic by-products that not only cause colon cancer but also damage the intestinal lining and make their way into the bloodstream, causing infection and many other age-related diseases (diabetes, autoimmunity, arthritis, and other chronic inflammatory disorders).[3]

You've no doubt heard that prescription antibiotics destroy "good" as well as harmful bacteria. It's less well known that significant amounts of antibiotics in milk, meat, and poultry do the same thing. When large numbers of good bacteria are destroyed, the consequent overgrowth of fungi, yeast, parasites, and dangerous bacteria can cause intestinal damage. Extensive damage leads to problems like ulcers, perforations, Crohn's disease, and ulcerative colitis. But far more common is a very insidious and often unsuspected condition in the gut (small and large intestines) known as "leaky gut syndrome."

Leaky Gut Syndrome

Leaky gut syndrome (LGS) is a chronic inflammatory process that increases the permeability of the intestines. Basically, the lining of the gut comes to resemble Swiss cheese. Food particles, harmful micro-organisms, and toxins easily make their way through these "leaks" and directly into the bloodstream. Since the barrier function of the intestines is compromised in LGS, the liver becomes overtaxed in its attempt to filter out this intestinal debris. As this debris makes its way into the bloodstream, the immune system is left to survey and sift through the waste. It, too, becomes exhausted, and immunity-related problems arise—allergies, chronic inflammatory conditions, and chronic or recurring infections.

Antibiotic-contaminated food and prescription antibiotics can contribute to LGS. Corticosteroid as well as nonsteroidal anti-inflammatory drugs, birth control pills, and hormone supplements can cause intestinal inflammation. Alcohol, caffeine, sugar, refined carbohydrates, food preservatives and dyes, wheat, and dairy proteins can cause imbalanced intestinal flora and chronic intestinal inflammation. Moreover, contaminated or heavily chlorinated water as well as all environmental toxins can lead to LGS. Chronic stress alone can make the gut permeable. Health problems associated with leaky gut syndrome include chronic fatigue, fibromyalgia, autoimmunity, and other chronic inflammatory conditions like asthma, arthritis, eczema, migraines, and psoriasis.[4]

With respect to nutrition, once LGS is established, optimal levels of protein, vitamins, minerals, and other essential nutrients can't get through the intestinal walls and into the bloodstream. This explains why some people continue to feel unwell despite an improved diet and additional nutritional supplements.

Systemic signs and symptoms of LGS are fatigue, chronic headache, lack of mental clarity, unexplained joint and muscular pain, and skin rashes. The more specific signs in the gut include excessive gas, chronic bloating, cramping pain, and irregular stools. When other intestinal diseases have been ruled out, LGS is often found to be the culprit. Towards the end of this chapter, we'll look at a program that helps combat LGS.

Elimination

In the last but not least phase of the digestive process, the large intestine propels waste forward for elimination. This phase, too, is critical for overall health. Bowel transit time is the time it takes for the waste from the food you eat to leave your system. In the North American population, this is anywhere from 48 to 72 hours, which is slow. On average, we consume less than 15 grams of fiber daily, which accounts for this poor bowel transit time. The high incidence of colorectal cancer, diverticulitis, and intestinal polyps in the aging North American population suggests that in this part of the world not enough fiber is being consumed and bowel transit time is too long.

The Role of Fiber

Both the Canadian Cancer Society and the U.S. National Cancer Institute recommend that you consume 40 grams of fiber daily. If you find it difficult to get this amount from whole grains, fruits, and vegetables alone, consider taking a powder fiber supplement. Ideal supplements are psyllium seed and husks, rice bran, oat bran, apple pectin, flaxseed, and guar gum, all of which contain both soluble and insoluble fibers.

Adequate fiber intake improves bowel transit time and helps lower cholesterol. High-fiber diets also slow down the rate that glucose enters the bloodstream and thereby help to keep blood-sugar levels steady. Fiber binds not only gut-derived toxins but also environmental toxins (including heavy metals) and pulls them out of the gut before they poison the body. Keep in mind that the fewer toxins from your gut that your liver has to deal with, the better it functions. Equally important, fiber promotes the growth of beneficial bacteria, strengthens the lining of the colon (thereby improving its function and keeping toxins from entering the bloodstream), and acidifies the colon (thus preventing the formation of toxins and harmful bacterial overgrowth).

Ideally, you should have at least one solid stool movement daily. Eating fiber-rich foods and drinking 6–8 glasses of pure water each day promote regular bowel movements. Adequate sleep, exercise, and the successful management of stress will also keep things moving. A regular routine, which means going to bed and waking up at the same time each day, helps to synchronize bowel function. Interestingly, food sensitivities, particularly cow's milk, can be major factors in chronic constipation.[5]

Now that you've had a fairly detailed look at the responsibilities of your digestive tract, let's sum it all up. A healthy gastrointestinal tract should do the following:

- Digest food properly
- Carry vitamins and minerals, proteins, essential fatty acids, and glucose across the gut lining into the bloodstream
- Participate in the continuous detoxification process needed for optimal health
- Act as the first line of defense to keep dangerous bacteria and toxins from slipping into the bloodstream
- Efficiently eliminate waste

Strategies for Better Digestive Health

The Basic Program

After age 40, there is a 20–30 percent decrease in the body's ability to produce digestive enzymes. And things get worse with aging. We propose seven simple things you can do to have better digestion and maintain a lifetime of health. By following these seven steps for at least three months, you will very likely not only improve your digestive powers, but also have greater and more sustainable energy levels.

Step 1   Eat at least three meals daily at consistent times. This will train your digestive system to have a natural rhythm. Don't let yourself get ravenous, but avoid large meals that put stress on your digestive system. Follow the Modified Elimination Diet outlined in Chapter 7, Appendix 7.2.

Step 2   Avoid drinking liquids during meals, as this dilutes and washes away digestive enzymes. Drink plenty of liquids (preferably at room temperature or hot) 30 minutes or so before meals to promote the flow of digestive juices. Wait for 15–30 minutes after meals before having liquids again.

Step 3   Allow enough time for your meals and chew your food thoroughly. Eat in a relaxed manner.

Step 4   To promote intestinal movement, start each and every day with 1–2 full glasses of water. It's also a good idea to squeeze half a fresh lemon into the water to alkalinize your system. Drink 6–8 glasses of pure water throughout the day.

Step 5   Add digestive enzymes to your meals. They may be taken at the beginning of the meal, during, or after. Choose a high-quality and well-balanced enzyme that aids in the digestion of proteins, fats, carbohydrates, and fiber. If you have an active or bleeding ulcer, avoid enzymes that contain hydrochloric acid or protease, as they can irritate the stomach lining. Do not take animal-derived enzymes for prolonged periods (more than six months), as they may reduce the production and secretion of your body's own enzymes. If you need enzyme supplements on an ongoing basis, choose plant-derived varieties (e.g., Organika's Full Spectrum Plant Enzymes®) that are active across a wide range of stomach pH. Also safe for long-term use, herbal bitters have a more far-reaching effect, since they stimulate secretions from the stomach, liver, gallbladder, pancreas, and intestines. Herbal bitters taken before meals stimulate appetite; taken 10–15 minutes after, they improve digestion, especially of fats. Those who have had their gallbladder removed should probably take them after a meal or avoid them altogether. The reason is that herbal bitters can stimulate a liver without a gallbladder to produce highly acidic bile that can irritate the intestines.

Step 6   Take beneficial bacterial supplements in the morning just before breakfast and before supper or at bedtime. Choose a high-quality, multi-strain bacterial supplement that has been prepared from non-dairy sources; these are generally better tolerated. Take these for at least six months to experience the full benefits.

Step 7 Add extra fiber to your daily regime, either in the morning or at bedtime. One of the best options is fresh-ground flaxseed; take 3 tablespoonsful or more daily. Psyllium seeds and husks ensure regularity. Apple and citrus pectin, as well as oat and rice bran, are great for lowering cholesterol and regulating blood sugar. If your bowels are sensitive, find fiber supplements that have marshmallow and/or slippery elm, as they are very soothing to irritated tissues. Ideally, try to get 10–20 grams (or more if well tolerated) in supplemental form on top of a high-fiber diet. First-time users should start with small amounts, then gradually increase the amount over a one- to two-week period. When using fiber in powder form, drink 1/3–1/2 teaspoon dissolved in water at a time. Those who find fiber powder unappealing can take capsules. Be sure that there are no added sugars or synthetic flavorings in your fiber supplements, and always store them in the refrigerator to ensure freshness.

The Importance of Cleansing and Detoxification

The above seven steps take us a certain distance on the road to better digestive health, but most of us should also go on a cleansing and detoxification program. Why? Because of our exposure to stress and to environmental toxins in the air, water, and food supply. Repeated cleansing helps to optimize health. Cleansing and detoxification programs are especially important for those who suffer from allergies, headaches, constipation, poor skin health, chronic inflammatory disorders, and weight problems.

Numerous cleansing and detoxification kits are available in health food stores and pharmacies. ReCleanse is a kit that has been clinically used for over 75 years by master herbalists at the Dominion Herbal College in Vancouver, B.C., the oldest and one of the most reputable schools in North America for the study of phytomedicines. The health principle behind ReCleanse is simple: regularly support your body in its natural elimination and detoxifying process and you will increasingly enable it to heal and function optimally; in this way, you will gradually achieve better health. The following is a list of some of the phytomedicines in ReCleanse:

- Buchu leaves: urinary tract cleanser, diuretic
- Juniper berries: eliminates uric acid, diuretic
- Cranberry extract: prevents urinary tract infections
- Uva ursi: soothes inflammation of bladder, kidneys, and prostate
- Cleavers: skin, blood, lymph, and urinary tract cleanser
- Dandelion root: cleanses liver and gallbladder, promotes digestion, diuretic
- Golden seal root: anti-microbial, digestive tonic, cleanses all mucous membranes
- Burdock root: cleanses blood, detoxifies lymphatic system
- Oregon grape root: anti-microbial, skin and blood cleanser
- Psyllium husk: cleanses intestinal tract; normalizes bowel function

- Slippery elm bark: cleanses mucus from bowels, soothes irritable and ulcerated bowels
- Norwegian kelp: eliminates toxins and heavy metals, excellent source of minerals

Ideally, cleansing should be done at least twice a year, spring and fall. Use ReCleanse or any other well-formulated cleansing and detoxification kit for one week to a month, depending on your level of commitment and experience. Another option is to use a kit of ReCleanse, which takes one week to complete, once a month until improvement in health occurs. You can follow the dietary guidelines for the ReCleanse program—see Appendix 7.1 for more information—or you can follow the Modified Elimination Diet (Chapter 7, Appendix 7.2) while you're on a cleansing program, to ensure its success.

You should expect to experience a few things while on a cleansing program. First, you'll urinate more and have more bowel movements. Second, you may develop cold- and flu-like symptoms. Finally, you may experience fatigue. All of these indicate that the body is being cleansed. Just be sure to drink 6–8 glasses of pure water daily to replace fluid loss and promote the excretions of toxins. If you experience significant fatigue, take electrolyte salts high in potassium and adaptogens to see your way through the cleansing process. Obviously, those who are critically ill, who take prescription medicines, or who have an acute infection, gallstones, or bowel obstruction should get clearance from their doctor before embarking on any cleansing program. The following is a list of the benefits of cleansing programs:

- Ability to cope better with stress
- Better sleep
- Clearer skin
- Control over inflammatory conditions
- Improved digestion and elimination
- Improved circulation and metabolism
- Mental clarity
- Stable blood sugar
- Sustained energy levels
- Weight loss

Why Cleansing Is Sometimes Not Enough

After following the seven steps for optimizing digestion and going on a cleansing and detoxification program, most people will have much better health. However, there are several reasons why some don't achieve optimal or sustainable wellness. For instance, individuals with mercury poisoning (most probably from dental fillings) would require a special detoxification program to regain their health. In addition, chronic infections caused by bacteria, parasites, and the surprisingly common fungus *Candida albicans* create specific intestinal and systemic problems that need to be addressed. A variety of phytomedicines have broad-spectrum activity against many tough-to-treat micro-organisms that manifest in different ways. The pesky *Candida albicans*, for example, can manifest as chronic fatigue and multiple food and environmental sensitivities. Take the survey in Appendix 9.1 to determine whether an overgrowth of the *Candida* fungus is a major factor for you. If your score is very high, you may want to add one or a combination of the following phytomedicines to your cleansing and detoxification program (all of these have an antibiotic-like effect on a variety of bacteria, fungi, parasites, and viruses): extracts of grapefruit seed, golden seal root, olive leaf, Oregon grape root, and oregano oil.[6]

Healing a Leaky Gut

Leaky gut syndrome, discussed earlier, keeps many people from achieving long-lasting health. The 4R Gastrointestinal Restoration Program devised by the Institute for Functional Medicine has been shown in clinical trials to help heal LGS. The benefits of this program include better digestive health, the easing (or curing) of chronic inflammatory disorders, and improved energy levels. This program optimizes the functioning of the intestinal immune system, which comprises nearly 70 percent of the body's total immune function. With the intestinal immune system providing a better first line of defense, more resilient health is created. See Appendix 9.2 for more information about the 4R program and to find out how to locate a practitioner in your area familiar with this approach.

Addressing Specific Gastrointestinal Problems

People suffering from either stomach or duodenal ulcers (collectively known as peptic ulcers) have numerous treatment options beyond what has already been mentioned. Depending on your particular situation, one or a combination of the following may prove invaluable in optimizing gastrointestinal health.

Deglycyrrhizinated Licorice (DGL)

DGL has been shown to heal peptic ulcers. Interestingly, DGL doesn't block the secretion or production of acid as conventional prescription medications and over-the-counter antacids do. Instead, it promotes blood circulation to the lining of the stomach and intestines, stimulates the production of new intestinal cells, and improves the quality of cells. While the prolonged use of licorice extracts can cause sodium retention and high blood pressure, this is not true of DGL, since the compounds in licorice responsible for these side effects have been removed from DGL.[7]

Mastica Gum

This resinous compound, derived from a tree that grows on the Greek island of Chios, has been shown to heal peptic ulcers. While the complete mechanism is not known, mastica gum does have antibacterial properties, in particular against one of the ulcer-causing bacteria. One of mastica gum's many advantages is that it doesn't disturb gastrointestinal flora as antibiotics typically do; therefore, if needed, it can be used on a long-term basis, unlike antibiotics.[8]

Ulcinex™

Ulcinex™ (the trade name of a product distributed by Metagenics) has been shown to be useful for heartburn, acid indigestion, upset stomach, and intestinal spasms. This multi-botanical formula also rebuilds intestinal tissue and destroys a variety of harmful bacteria. Moreover, Ulcinex™ protects the gut from stress, overproduction of acids, and irritants such as alcohol and coffee.[9]

Aloe Vera Gel, Marshmallow Root, and Slippery Elm Bark

All these substances contain mucopolysaccharides, gooey compounds that help soothe and heal irritated or ulcerated gastrointestinal tissues. These compounds actually adhere to the site of injury and protect the tissue from acids, bacteria, and other irritants until the damage can be repaired.[10]

Cardamom, Chamomile, Fennel, Ginger, Peppermint, Rosemary, and Thyme

These herbs are some natural choices that help to improve digestion and elimination, break up gas, stop intestinal spasms, offer pain relief, and control inflammation. They can be used to treat the symptoms of irritable bowel syndrome, ulcerative colitis, and Crohn's disease.[11]

Colostrum

Colostrum is a collection of biological proteins derived from the first few days of milk secretion from cows that have just delivered. Highly purified colostrums don't contain appreciable amounts of casein (the major milk protein) or lactose (milk sugar) and are thus well tolerated by those with dairy allergies or intolerances. Colostrum works with the intestinal immune system to destroy intestinal bugs and helps to heal gut damage. It is useful in treating diarrhea brought on by harmful micro-organisms and in healing ulcers, inflammatory bowel diseases, and leaky gut syndrome.[12] Take high-quality colostrum for several months to get its benefit.

Conclusion

The purpose of this chapter has been to describe the duties of the digestive tract and the challenges it faces throughout a lifetime. People of every age experience better health by optimizing digestion. The basic program for digestive health plus routine cleansing is often enough to bring the gut back into shape. Some may need to go further, especially those with digestive diseases and disorders. The payoff in going these extra distances is better overall health and improved chances for healthy aging. It is becoming increasingly clear that your vitality, physical appearance, and mental clarity all pivot on a well-tuned gut.

10

CHRONIC INFLAMMATION AND AGING

We will now discuss how and why inflammation becomes chronic. This is a highly relevant topic, since if inflammation goes uncontrolled, aging accelerates and a variety of chronic diseases and conditions develop. This chapter provides strategies to prevent and treat this pernicious process.

Let's begin by asking what the following age-related diseases and conditions have in common:

- Allergies
- Asthma
- Autoimmunity
- Cancer
- Cardiovascular disease
- Eczema
- Endometriosis
- Migraines

- Fibromyalgia
- Irritable bowel syndrome
- Macular degeneration
- Osteoarthritis
- Peptic ulcer
- Psoriasis
- Sinusitis
- Ulcerative colitis

If your answer was that all these situations involve a chronic inflammatory process, you're right. In fact, aging itself can be thought of as a loss of inflammatory control that leads to cellular destruction and loss of function. The increasing pain and fatigue most of us experience as we grow older is due to chronic systemic inflammation.[1]

Inflammation: Its Symptoms and Purpose

In the case of localized inflammation (i.e., inflammation in response to injury), the symptoms of redness, heat, pain, and swelling encourage us to protect the injury and give it time to heal. In the case of infection, inflammation is set in motion to prevent the attacking microbes from spreading into healthy tissue. Fever is sometimes produced to help the body better deal with infectious germs. Acute inflammation—either from physical trauma or infection—is a destructive process, but it is the body's way of removing damaged cells and debris so that the healing process can take place. When the immune system is functioning properly, repair is successful and the inflammatory process will have been a limited phenomenon.

Why Inflammation Becomes Chronic

Unfortunately, there is not always a happy ending. A variety of factors can make inflammation chronic. The inflammatory process creates excessive numbers of free radicals, and when these are not sufficiently buffered, they go on to damage healthy cells; reciprocally, the surplus of free radicals can incite the inflammatory process, completing the vicious circle. A diet high in vitamins C, E, beta carotene, and other plant compounds obtained from whole grains, fruits, and vegetables helps to staunch excessive free-radical production. On the other hand, a diet high in calories, animal protein, saturated fat, sugar, refined carbohydrates, and salt perpetuates the inflammatory process once it's engaged. The latter diet spells a delayed recovery from sickness and injury, and when the inflammatory process runs on longer than it should, healthy tissue is needlessly destroyed. Chronic inflammation also finds a home in sufferers of leaky gut syndrome (see Chapter 9), since gut-derived toxins, micro-organisms, and undigested food particles slip easily into the bloodstream to trigger inflammation. The overload of environmental allergens, chemicals, and toxins can also ignite the inflammatory process.

Beyond poor nutrition, poor intestinal tract integrity, and inefficient detoxification, certain lifestyle factors also determine the duration of inflammation. Prolonged stress, insufficient rest and relaxation, not enough water, smoking, and too much caffeine and alcohol can individually or collectively make it hard for the body to shut down inflammation. The misuse or overuse of antihistamines, antibiotics, steroids, and non-steroidal anti-inflammatory (NSAIDs) medications can also create imbalances in the inflammatory process.

How Inflammation Becomes Chronic

To understand how inflammation becomes chronic, we need to understand how the body tries to keep the inflammatory process balanced. Three essential fatty acids (arachidonic, omega-6, and omega-3) are incorporated into your cell membranes to provide structural integrity and flexibility. They are converted into hormone-like compounds, known as *eicosanoids*. The ratio of these three major fatty acids within your cell membranes determines the extent and duration of inflammation. It is important to know that the dietary sources of omega-6, omega-3, and arachidonic acid can lead to either anti-inflammatory or inflammatory eicosanoid chemicals. Furthermore, some critical nutrients are needed to convert the dietary sources of omega-6 and omega-3 into their respective anti-inflammatory chemicals. When your cell membranes are dominated by the arachidonic fatty acid, inflammation and free-radical damage flare up like a blazing forest fire, and as cell membranes are saturated with this type of fat, they become stiff and don't allow nutrients to readily flow inside the cell and waste to be pumped out. Table 10.1 presents a summary of the major functions of eicosanoids.

TABLE 10.1: Functions of Eicosanoids Derived from the Omega-6 and Omega-3 Fatty Acids and from Arachidonic Acid

FUNCTIONS OF EICOSANOIDS DERIVED FROM
THE OMEGA-6 AND OMEGA-3 FATTY ACIDS

Anti-inflammatory	Improve red blood cell flexibility
Control pain	Improve immune function
Decrease blood pressure	Control cell proliferation
Increase calibre of blood vessels and	Regulate blood sugar
Improve circulation	Balance hormones
Inhibit cholesterol synthesis	Improve organ and glandular function (espe-
Protect lining of stomach	cially brain, heart, liver, kidney, adrenals,
Prevent platelet aggregation and clotting	gut)

FUNCTIONS OF EICOSANOIDS DERIVED FROM ARACHIDONIC ACID

Decrease the calibre of blood vessels and circulation	Increase blood pressure
Increase pain and inflammation	Increase platelet aggregation and clotting
Increase sodium and water retention	Depresse immune function
	Increase cell proliferation

What you need to appreciate is that the inflammatory eicosanoids must be balanced by the anti-inflammatory eicosanoids. If your diet is rich in whole grains, fruits, and vegetables (especially leafy greens) and you have a balanced intake of lean animal protein (fish, chicken, turkey, beef, eggs) and vegetable protein (rice, soy, beans, nuts, seeds), you can assume that you're taking in a balanced amount of the three major dietary fatty acids. Such a diet would promote balanced inflammatory processes.

When you consume a lot of red meat (beef and pork), eggs, milk, cheese, ice cream, and peanuts, all high in arachidonic acid and trans fatty acids (margarine and snack foods), your body overproduces dangerous inflammatory chemicals. Furthermore, stress, alcohol, caffeine, sugar, refined carbohydrates, and various nutrient insufficiencies inhibit the production of the body's own natural anti-inflammatory chemicals.

During the aging process, there is a decline in beneficial eicosanoids and a rise in the harmful eicosanoids. When the production of the harmful eicosanoids is unimpeded, numerous age-related chronic inflammatory diseases and conditions can develop. These include high blood pressure, heart disease, cancer, diabetes, arthritis, and weight gain.

Controlling Inflammation with Essential Fatty Acids

Fortunately, the process of chronic inflammation is the same whatever its location. It doesn't matter whether you're dealing with heart disease, arthritis, asthma, or even migraines—they are all chronic inflammatory disorders and they all involve imbalances in the essential fatty acids. Supplementing with the essential omega-6 and omega-3 fatty acids helps the body produce its own anti-inflammatory chemicals and thereby better contend with chronic inflammation. Table 10.2 shows some of the different conditions treated by and different benefits of the omega-6 (evening primrose) and omega-3 (flaxseed oil and fish oil) fatty acids:[2]

TABLE 10.2: Conditions Treated by and Benefits of the Omega-6 and Omega-3 Fatty Acids

CONDITIONS	BENEFITS
Acne	Enhance energy levels and improve endurance
Allergies	Enhance fertility (both men and women)
Arthritis	Ensure proper growth and development
Asthma	Improve brain function and mood
Autoimmunity	Improve circulation
Cancer	Improve digestion and elimination
Cardiovascular disease	Improve immune function
Diabetes	Improve kidney functioning
Dry eyes, hair, and skin	Improve motor coordination
Eczema	Improve tissue oxygenation
Hair loss	Improve tooth and bone health
Hyperactivity	Improve vision and learning
Hypertension	Lower cholesterol and triglycerides
Menopause	Raise HDL (good cholesterol)
Multiple sclerosis	
Neuropathy	
Obesity	
Pre-menstrual syndrome	
Psoriasis	

When balanced in the body, the essential fatty acids improve cell-membrane fluidity. When cell membranes are more fluid, hormones and neurotransmitters bind to cells and work better. Thus, insulin is better able to regulate blood sugar, and serotonin is better able to regulate mood and sleep. Furthermore, when membranes are fluid, nutrients are more easily transported inside the cell and waste can be more efficiently pumped out. In other words, essential fatty acids improve cellular traffic and thus enhance overall health.

Taking Action to Control Inflammation

At this point, let's lay out a plan of action to control aging, age-related diseases, and all chronic inflammatory disorders.

1. Identify the sources of stress in your life and develop better coping strategies. Refer back to Chapter 3 and go over what robs you of good health. Review Chapter 5 for guidelines on how to create emotional balance. Then check Chapter 8 for information on how nutrition and dietary supplements can help you deal with stress.

2. Take a good look at your diet. Identify food sensitivities by following the Elimination Diet outlined in Chapter 7. Completely eliminate trans fatty acids, refined carbohydrates, sugar, and alcohol. If possible, kick the caffeine habit or have no more than two cups of coffee daily. Increase dietary intake of omega-3 fatty acids by eating cold-water fish and flaxseeds. You can also purchase eggs, whole grain cereals, and breads high in omega-3 fatty acids.

3. Identify any signs and symptoms of poor gastrointestinal function and follow the suggestions to improve digestion in Chapter 9; consider following a detoxification and cleansing program. Remember that intestinal contents can sometimes make their way into the bloodstream and trigger inflammation. Therefore, if you have a chronic inflammatory disorder, you'd do well to start your investigation with the gut.

4. Take a high-quality, well-balanced multiple vitamin and mineral supplement (unless there is a need, preferably without iron) with each meal. Also add 400–800 IU of natural mixed vitamin E and 500–3,000 milligrams of vitamin C daily. Doing this will provide the micronutrients needed to help convert the essential fatty acids into the beneficial anti-inflammatory chemicals. Also, vitamins E and C help control the damaging effects of free radicals created by inflammation.

5. Take 1–2 tablespoons of Udo's Choice Ultimate Oil Blend on a daily basis. Taking this oil is one of the best ways to get a good balance of omega-6 and omega-3 fatty acids. One to 2 tablespoons of this oil blend added to 2 scoops of UltraInflamX™ by Metagenics (known as UltraInflavogen in Canada) can be used as a meal replacement or taken between meals one to three times daily. UltraInflamX™ is a hypoallergenic rice-

protein medical food that contains vitamins, minerals, and phytomedicines to control all chronic inflammatory disorders.

6. Take a super green food drink daily. Super green foods are combinations of plants from the sea (blue green algae, chlorella) and land (wheat grass, barley grass, alfalfa) that are high in chlorophyll and rich in minerals. They're excellent to take on a daily basis because they help neutralize free radicals and metabolic acids, common features in aging and all chronic inflammatory disorders. Your blood and tissues should have a pH of 7.35 to 7.40 (slightly alkaline), as the body functions optimally in this range. These super green foods help the body maintain a desirable alkaline pH. Greens+™ (manufactured by Ehn) is a good choice, and you can add Udo's Oil alone or Udo's Oil plus the UltraInflamX™ to create an exceptionally nutrient-dense drink.

When followed for at least three months, these six steps greatly alleviate any chronic inflammatory disorder. Besides feeling less pain, you will probably have more sustainable energy and be better able to deal with stress.

We'll now move on to explore treatment options for specific chronic inflammatory disorders. You can expand on the six-step plan above by adding the options that apply to you. Those of you on blood-thinning medications or with bleeding disorders should get clearance from your doctor before proceeding.

Arthritis

Osteoarthritis is an age-related condition involving wear and tear of the connective tissue (mostly cartilage) that typically affects the knees, hips, and spinal joints. Non-steroidal anti-inflammatory drugs (NSAIDs) are commonly prescribed for arthritis. However, the evidence shows that daily long-term use (months to years) of NSAIDs accelerates the degenerative process in osteoarthritis. It appears that NSAIDs prevent the formation of new cartilage tissue, accelerate the destruction of already damaged cartilage, and destroy healthy cartilage tissue.[3] As well, NSAIDs may increase gut permeability; leaky gut syndrome (LGS), which fuels the inflammatory process, could be the result.[4] Long-term NSAIDs may have other side effects as well, including gastrointestinal ulcers, sodium and water retention, high blood pressure, and poor immune function.

The basic problem is that all anti-inflammatory medications block both inflammatory and anti-inflammatory pathways in the body. When the body's inherent mechanisms for controlling inflammation are suppressed, the healing of damaged tissue cannot take place. Therefore, the long-term use of NSAIDs should be avoided.

Glucosamine Sulfate

Glucosamine sulfate has become a very popular and safe nutritional supplement for arthritis sufferers. This compound has been shown to stimulate the production of new cartilage tissue and block destructive enzymes that break down connective tissue. As well, glucosamine sulfate incorporates itself into existing cartilage tissue and draws water there to provide better cushioning and shock absorption. Its action is threefold: it acts as a very safe anti-inflammatory (albeit mild) and improves both the quality and quantity of connective tissue, especially cartilage.[5]

"How much should I consider taking?" It is recommended that people with osteoarthritis who weigh less than 150 pounds take 1,500 milligrams of glucosamine sulfate daily, either all at once or in divided doses; those over 150 pounds should take 2,000–3,000 milligrams daily. Patience is needed, as it can take months for results to be realized.

"What is the best form of glucosamine?" Glucosamine sulfate is the most widely studied and accepted form. One of the best available is GLS® 500 by Organika. It contains 500 milligrams of sodium-free glucosamine sulfate per capsule, making it safe for people on salt-restricted diets. GLS® 500 was one of the first glucosamine sulfate products on the market; available for over 10 years, it has been time-tested and proven to help most of those who suffer from osteoarthritis. (See Appendix 7.1.)

"Should I take chondroitin sulfate along with glucosamine sulfate?" The information on chondroitin sulfate isn't as abundant as that on glucosamine sulfate, but the anecdotal evidence that does exist suggests that when chondroitin is taken with glucosamine, good results are achieved in most cases. There are therefore those who believe that this combination works best. This may be true, but without hard evidence, it's difficult to say whether chondroitin is essential. One drawback to adding chondroitin is its cost. Should you decide to add it, take 400 milligrams of chondroitin (preferably at 90 percent concentration) for every 500 milligrams of glucosamine. Once again, be patient, as it can be months before results are achieved.

"Can I take glucosamine sulfate if I have allergies or severe reactions to sulfa-based prescription medications?" The sulfate found in glucosamine occurs naturally in the body and is unrelated to sulfa-based drugs. There have never been any reports of an allergic reaction to glucosamine sulfate. It can therefore be safely taken even by those with sulfa-based drug allergies. In a very small percentage of the population, glucosamine sulfate can cause mild stomach discomfort. Those with sensitive stomachs are thus advised to take it with meals.

"What are some safe alternatives to NSAIDs that I can take on a daily basis to control the pain and decrease the inflammation of my osteoarthritis and improve joint mobility?" *Ginger root extract* can be used daily to control the pain and inflammation of arthritis. Ginger is also a potent antioxidant, as it neutralizes free radicals. Moreover, it improves digestion and prevents blood clots, thereby improving circulation and controlling systemic inflammation. In fact, 500 compounds identified in ginger root extract together have a broad spectrum of activity against the many mechanisms of inflammation.[6]

Bromelain, an enzyme derived from pineapples, not only blocks the production of inflammatory chemicals but also helps the body produce its own anti-inflammatory chemicals. As well, bromelain helps to break down scar tissue and adhesions and other consequences of inflammation that decrease mobility and increase swelling. Therefore, bromelain can be used for painful, hot, stiff, and swollen joints. It also aids in the digestion of protein-rich foods, cuts down on allergic reactions, helps heal the gut, and regulates the circulatory system.[7]

Curcumin, a yellow compound derived from the turmeric root and used as a spice in many Indian dishes, has potent anti-inflammatory and antioxidant properties. It modulates the immune system by decreasing the production of chemicals that trigger inflammation. It also protects and improves liver function. Specifically, curcumin improves bile flow from the liver, thereby lowering cholesterol levels and removing toxins from the system. Look for curcumin standardized at 95 percent curcuminoids (the active components); it combines well with bromelain to control acute pain and inflammation from flare-ups.[8]

Asthma and Allergies

We'll talk about asthma and allergies together because they are interconnected through chronic inflammation. Asthma can be induced by infection, exercise, stress, and smoking. A large percentage of asthmatics, however, have several environmental allergies and food sensitivities. Thus, asthma can be seen as an allergic reaction localized in the lungs. Allergic reactions can occur anywhere in the body, and in the case of seasonal allergies, they often manifest in the eyes, sinuses, throat, and lungs.

A word of caution for unstable asthmatics who rely on inhalers: because of the potential seriousness of asthma attacks, never *replace* your inhaler with any of the remedies that we will be suggesting below. All these suggestions, as well as the others made throughout this chapter, can be used alongside your inhaler. You may find, however, that over time you'll have a decreased need for your inhaler and may even be able to get off it altogether with the supervision of your doctor. Inquire about purchasing a peak flow meter to monitor improvements in lung function.

Quercetin is a natural plant compound found in high amounts in tea, onions, garlic, and many fruits and vegetables. It has anti-inflammatory, antioxidant properties and stabilizes certain cells of the immune system to prevent the release of excessive amounts of histamine. Quercetin is thus ideal for preventing and managing allergies and asthma. Adding grape seed extract to quercetin can boost its activity, offering greater control of allergic reactions. Adding bromelain can help break congestion in the upper and lower respiratory tract.[9]

Stinging nettle, a natural plant extract rich in vitamin C and minerals, has anti-inflammatory, antioxidant, anti-allergy, and immune-modulating properties. With regular use, stinging nettle controls the frequency and intensity of allergies.[10]

The phytomedicine *ginkgo biloba* helps to regulate circulation, but it also has anti-inflammatory and antioxidant properties. Adult sufferers of asthma may find standardized extract of ginkgo biloba ideal because it can help dilate the bronchial tubes, control inflammation in lungs, and improve circulation to the lungs. This phytomedicine does not deal with the acute symptoms of asthma and may provide benefit only when taken regularly.[11]

Forskolin is a phytomedicine with similar properties to ginkgo biloba in that it can be used regularly for the better management of asthma in adults. However, it also improves digestion, promotes weight loss, and lowers high blood pressure. Thus, forskolin is preferred over ginkgo in the treatment of asthma when these other problems exist.[12]

Migraines

Migraine sufferers, like all sufferers of chronic inflammatory disorders, should try to identify foods that act as triggers. A migraine attack can be viewed as an inflammatory reaction that happens in the circulatory system. Platelets aggregate in the blood vessels of the brain and release inflammatory chemicals that cause extreme dilation of the blood vessels. Swelling, pain, and pressure in the head occur because of the dilation. Nausea and heightened sensitivity to light and noise also accompany migraine attacks.

Feverfew, taken on a regular basis, helps to control the inflammatory process and stabilizes platelets seen in migraines. Should you decide to try feverfew, select a high-quality standardized extract and keep it refrigerated to prevent the volatile oils in this plant compound from oxidizing. Feverfew should be taken daily for a three- to four-month period before any benefit can be seen. After this length of time, discontinue for four weeks and then resume if there is still a need or if benefit was experienced. Feverfew must be used in this fashion and is of little value in the management of acute migraine attacks.

Ginger root extract can prove to be quite useful as an acute remedy for migraine attacks, as it is a natural pain reliever and settles nausea.[13]

Fibromyalgia

Fibromyalgia is an inflammatory disorder of the muscles that involves pain and weakness throughout most of the body. Typically, it also involves chronic fatigue. Patients with fibromyalgia experience digestive problems, poor mental function, depression, and sleeping disorders, all of which can be debilitating. People diagnosed with fibromyalgia or chronic fatigue syndrome may try combinations of *ginger, curcumin,* and *bromelain* in addition to the six nutritional steps outlined earlier that help to control inflammation and improve energy levels.

When prescription medicines fail and nutritional interventions only temporarily help, it is best to seek guidance from a health practitioner experienced with complex inflammatory disorders. The Institute for Functional Medicine (800-228-0622; Gig Harbor, Washington, U.S.A.) could help you locate a specialist in chronic inflammatory disorders in your area of North America.

Conclusion

This chapter will have helped you appreciate that there are multiple causes of chronic inflammation and that anti-inflammatory mechanisms within the body can be nutritionally supported. To give your body support, you first need to make changes in your diet and lifestyle. Then you can choose among the many naturally derived compounds capable of controlling inflammation and supporting the body's own anti-inflammatory mechanisms.

Aging, age-related diseases, and chronic disorders all involve chronic inflammation gone unchecked. The suggestions outlined in this chapter offer a comprehensive approach. It requires effort and patience on your part before benefits are realized. Remember that sometimes pain is unavoidable. However, better food choices and recent discoveries from our plant kingdom now make most suffering optional.

11

SHIELDS FOR THE IMMUNE SYSTEM

A properly functioning immune system is essential for health and longevity. It is the main defense in the battle against infection, environmental poisons, potential cellular decay, and cancer. If it becomes weakened or unbalanced, problems can arise. An underactive immune system can result in serious infections and even organ damage. An overactive system can lead to autoimmune disorders, such as rheumatoid arthritis and lupus.

As people age, their immune system can become less efficient in battling intruders; it might even target healthy cells—as is the case with autoimmune disorders. If you take the time to understand the lines of defense the immune system provides, you can better prepare, through diet and lifestyle, for a lifetime of warfare against intruding organisms. When the body's natural defenses are not enough on their own, there are plenty of immune system reinforcements—vitamins, minerals, plant-source products, and other nutritional supplements—that you can call upon to give yourself a boost.

Your Great Defender

When the immune system jumps into action, it can use a variety of organs and cells to respond to the offender. The body has general barriers of protection—the mucous lining of the nasal passages and mouth, for example—that trap bacteria. There are also specific responses—antibody-mediated or cell-mediated pathways—that can distinguish foreign molecules or damaged self-molecules (molecules from within the body) from healthy self-molecules. It's important to understand how all this works.

Cell-Mediated Immunity

The lymphatic system produces the cells for the immune system, and once matured, these cells can be found in any tissue, identifying potential invaders and removing damaged cells. This remarkable system is composed of lymph vessels, lymph nodes, bone marrow, and the thymus gland. The lymph vessels and lymph nodes are used to absorb excess fluid to be returned to the blood and are therefore very important for proper circulation. Special lymph cells called *lymphocytes* are produced in the bone marrow; as they mature, they differentiate into B and T cells.

The thymus is the master gland of the immune system. It produces several hormones, including *thymosin*, which stimulates the lymphocytes to mature into T cells. These T cells control cell-mediated immunity by helping to activate cells that identify invaders (bacteria, viruses) as "non-self" cells and destroy them.

Antibody-Mediated Immunity

B cells are involved in antibody-mediated immune response, as they produce and release antibodies. Antibodies identify foreign proteins (antigens), bind to them, and replicate to create more cells to respond to the invaders. B cells also become memory cells, so that each time you are exposed to a specific infectious organism or chemical the response time is reduced and your body can fight the offender more efficiently. This is why allergic reactions to certain chemicals have a faster onset and are more severe with each exposure.

It's amazing how the body responds to foreign invaders when it is functioning optimally. *Macrophages* (a type of immune cell) come along and engulf the "bad guys" (such as a virus or chemical) and then display on their cell wall fragments of the protein, thus identifying the invader. This alerts the B and T cells to respond. Thus begins the war against the invader.

Immune responses can also be triggered outside the lymphatic system. Certain tissues (called *mucosal associated lymphoid tissue*, or MALT) contain combinations of macrophages and various types of lymphocytes present in the digestive, respiratory, and urogenital systems. Again, the function of these cells is to identify and eliminate invaders. For an example, let's look at the immune functions of the digestive system. As you eat a meal, the food passes through the mouth, esophagus, stomach, and so on. As it goes down, the food comes across different areas of this specific tissue (in the digestive system it's called GALT—*gut associated lymphoid tissue*), and the lymphocytes and macrophages can sift through it to identify any foreign substances or cells; this is similar to the action in the lymphatic system. The lymphocyte and macrophage cells remove the offenders by transporting them to the nearest lymph node and on through the lymphatic system.

Aging and Immunity

As we age, the efficiency of the immune system decreases. Older adults are at a greater risk of infection, and when it occurs, it takes them longer to heal and the consequences can be more serious. Older adults also have a diminished response to chemicals produced by the immune system when it's fighting infection. For example, a serious infection may not produce a fever and may thus go undetected longer.

Why does immunity decline with aging? There are a number of reasons. Older adults have the same number of lymphocytes as younger adults, but these cells are less likely to react to foreign substances. As we age, the thymus shrinks in size and becomes nearly dormant. Hormones also play a role. Elevated levels of stress hormones, such as cortisol, inhibit the immune response. Autoimmune responses also increase with age, causing the body to attack its own cells (as in rheumatoid arthritis and atherosclerosis). Vaccinations are often recommended for the elderly because of their impaired ability to fight off infections, yet vaccines are less effective in these people. Overall, seniors have a higher risk of developing serious infections and have longer recovery times.

Boosting the Immune System

While immune function usually declines with age, it doesn't have to. Good nutrition, regular and moderate exercise, stress management, and adequate sleep will support the immune system and keep it working efficiently.

Nutritional Strategies

It is well known that nutrition affects our immune system health. In fact, several indices of immune system health (antibody production, lymphocyte production, and numbers of immune cells) are influenced by nutrient intake. A diet rich in fruits, vegetables, beans, and legumes provides your body and immune system with the nutrients necessary for optimal functioning.

Water, too, can help improve your defenses. The mucous membranes (in the nose, eyes, and mouth) act as a physical barrier and are the first defense against invaders. Immune factors in body fluids coat the mucous membranes and offer protection. Allowing these areas to become dry or cracked is like opening the door to invaders; keeping them well hydrated by drinking plenty of water is one of the easiest and most effective ways to fight infection.

Green Foods

Since healthy eating is not always easy and practical, "green drinks or "super foods" have become a popular way to make up for nutritional shortcomings. These concoctions contain vitamins and minerals, vegetable and fruit powders, sprouted grains, algae, probi-otics (the health-promoting "friendly/good" bacteria), and digestive enzymes. Green drinks support immune function, improve digestion and detoxification, and improve energy and well-being. The many brands available vary in quality and formulation. We highly recommend Greens+, which can be found in health food stores and pharmacies throughout North America.

Diet and Immunity

Here are some other facts about diet and immunity to keep in mind:

- Diets high in refined sugar reduce immune function and increase the risk of infec-tion. Conversely, diets low in sugar help to improve immune function. Sugar (even honey) can hamper immune function by interfering with the ability of white blood cells to destroy bacteria.[1]
- It has been shown that too much dietary fat impairs the immune response. Reducing the amount of fat in your diet will enhance several indices of immune response.[2]
- Too much alcohol, even a single binge, can have a negative impact on your immune system, suppressing its function.[3]

The message is clear: go light on sugar and fat, consume alcohol in moderation, drink a lot of purified water, and follow a healthy diet.

Lifestyle Tips

Maintaining a healthy body weight is another important factor in maintaining immune function. Studies have shown that being either overweight or underweight can impair your immune responses.[4] Regular physical activity and exercise is a great way to strengthen the immune system and reduce the risk of infections.[5]

Chronic emotional and physical stress is a strong depressant of the immune system, increasing the risk of infections and even cancer.[6] Chronic stress elevates cortisol, causing a reduction in the hormone DHEA (dehydroepiandrosterone), and a lower level of DHEA reduces immune function. Proper nutrition and supplements combat the harmful effects of stress and improve immune function. Stress-reducing techniques such as relaxation exercises, meditation, and biofeedback can also improve immune function.[7] Review the information on how to beat stress in Chapter 5.

Nutritional Supplements and Immune Function

We have discussed the importance of a healthy diet for immunity, but diet alone may not be enough to protect us. For certain segments of the population—the elderly, smokers, those with poor diets (nutrient deficiencies), and those at increased risk of infection—the immune response can be increased through nutritional supplements.[8] Nutrients known to support and enhance immune function include beta carotene, vitamins A, C, E, and B12, glutathione, and zinc.

Vitamin A and Beta Carotene

Vitamin A has long been known to support immune function by helping the mucous membranes resist infection.[9] Beta carotene (pro-vitamin A) offers immune benefits by increasing immune cell numbers and activity. Research has shown immune benefits with beta carotene supplements in healthy people at 25,000–100,000 IU per day.[10] In the elderly, doses of 40,000–150,000 IU per day have increased the activity of the "natural killer" (NK) immune cells.[11]

Vitamin C

Vitamin C is popular for its immune-boosting activity. It appears to work by elevating the levels and enhancing the activity of certain immune cells, such as interferon.[12] Vitamin C is promoted to prevent colds, but the evidence is conflicting. A review of 20 studies concluded that up to several grams of vitamin C per day has only a small effect in preventing colds. Its benefits when taken at the onset of a cold are more significant, reducing the duration by an average of 23 percent.[13]

High doses of vitamin C (more than 1 gram per day) may cause diarrhea in some people. Many drugs, including oral contraceptives, indomethacin, corticosteroids, and Aspirin, deplete vitamin C levels. If you have a history of kidney stones, kidney failure, or hemachromatosis, consult your doctor before supplementing with vitamin C.

Vitamin E

Vitamin E is a well-known supportive nutrient for immune system health. At dosages greater than 200 IU daily, it has been shown to boost immune cell activity in the elderly.[14] The natural form of vitamin E (d-alpha tocopherol) is the preferred supplement, since it has greater antioxidant activity and absorption. Some cholesterol-lowering drugs (gemfi-brozil and bile-acid sequestrants) can weaken absorption of vitamin E. Those taking blood-thinning drugs such as warfarin should be aware that high doses of vitamin E (>1,200 IU daily) may enhance the drugs' anticoagulant effects.[15]

Vitamin B12

A deficiency of vitamin B12 has been linked to decreased immune function.[16] At particular risk of B12 deficiency are vegans, the elderly, those with malabsorption conditions (such as celiac disease), and those taking drugs that interfere with B12 absorption (oral contraceptives, anticonvulsants, erythromycin, tetracycline, and histamine blockers).[17] Recommended dosages of vitamin B12 vary greatly, from 3 micrograms per day for vegans, to 10–25 micrograms for the elderly, to as much as 1,000 micrograms daily for those with pernicious anemia.

Glutathione

This potent antioxidant is one of the most important supporters of immune function. It is produced by the body from other antioxidants and can be found in various fruits and vegetables. Glutathione is required for production of the T and B lymphocytes and helps the T-helper cells (Th-1) fight bacteria, viruses, and cancer. It also plays a role in controlling allergic reactions and inflammation. Supplements of glutathione are not very well absorbed; a better way to boost glutathione levels is through antioxidant supplements (such as lipoic acid) that provide the building blocks the body needs to make glutathione.

Zinc

Zinc is beneficial for wound healing and boosting immunity. Supplements of zinc have been reported to increase immune function and to shorten the duration and severity of the common cold.[18] Zinc is sometimes used as a preventive supplement for those experiencing recurrent infections. It is very safe at dosages below 50 milligrams. Avoid high doses (300 milligrams per day), as these may actually impair immune function.[19] Possible side effects include stomach ache, nausea, mouth irritation, and a metallic taste.

Antioxidant Combinations

Many researchers, including internationally known Dr. Lester Packer, feel that antioxidants work best in combination. Packer's "Network Antioxidants" include coenzyme Q10, vitamins C and E, glutathione, and lipoic acid. In researching these antioxidants, Dr. Packer found that they can enhance the power of each other (synergy) and are capable of recycling each other. This offers better protection against free radicals. Antioxidant blends are therefore preferred as an effective way to get full free-radical protection. Protect+™ by greens+™ Canada contains the network antioxidant blend.

Immune-Modulating Herbs

Panax Ginseng

Components of panax (Asian) ginseng are known to support immune function, counter the effects of stress, and reduce fatigue. One hundred milligrams of a standardized extract of Panax Ginseng C.A. Meyer twice daily was shown to improve immune function and reduce the incidence of colds and flus.[20] Asian ginseng is well tolerated by most individuals but may cause insomnia and increased blood pressure in some. It should be avoided in pregnancy and during lactation.

Echinacea

Echinacea stimulates the function of various immune cells, particularly natural killer cells, lymphocytes, and macrophages, and increases interferon production.[21] It also reduces the duration and severity of cold and flu symptoms.[22] While echinacea is often used for the prevention of infection, studies have yielded conflicting results.[23] The strongest evidence supports echinacea's use at the onset of infection. The usual dosage is 250–500 milligrams three times daily for 10 to 14 days. Echinacea is very safe and well tolerated, but it should be avoided by people with allergies to flowers in the daisy family.

Other Immune System Boosters

Probiotics

Commonly referred to as "friendly" bacteria, probiotic organisms such as *lactobacillus acidophilus* and *bifidobacterium bifidum* aid the immune system by inhibiting the growth of pathogenic (harmful) bacteria, boosting immune function, and increasing resistance to infection.[24] Probiotic bacteria produce compounds (lactic acid and hydrogen peroxide) that increase the acidity of the intestine and inhibit the growth of pathogenic bacteria. They also produce substances called bacteriocins, which function as natural antibiotics.[25] Many practitioners recommend probiotics during and after antibiotic treatments to replace the beneficial bacteria and restore the health of the intestine. A secondary effect of probiotics is the production of the B vitamins—niacin, folic acid, biotin, and vitamin B6.

The recommended dose depends on the strain used and the concentration of viable organisms, but it's usually 1–2 billion CFUs (colony-forming units) daily. Products vary greatly in quality and stability; many require refrigeration. We recommend Kyo-Dophilus by Wakunaga. Adverse reactions (upset stomach, gas) are minor and rare.

Thymus Extracts

The thymus gland plays an important role in immune function, including in the production of T lymphocytes. Thymus extracts have been shown to reduce the number of infections in children and adults with a history of recurrent respiratory tract infection.[26] They also improve immune function in diabetics, the elderly, and those with exercise-induced immune suppression.[27] Dosage varies according to the type of product used. There are no known side effects or drug interactions with thymus extracts.

Colostrum

Colostrum is the fluid produced by a mother cow's mammary glands just after delivery, before the onset of lactation. It is a rich source of vitamins, essential fatty acids, and various immune factors that nourish the newborn infant. Therapeutically, colostrum is derived from bovine sources and is used as a supplement to help strengthen the immune system, promote wound healing, and treat stomach disorders.

Plant Sterols and Sterolins

Sterols and sterolins are plant nutrients (they occur naturally in fruits, vegetables, seeds, and nuts) that have the ability to activate immune cells that modulate immunity. They are useful for both overactive and underactive immune systems.

Since these plant compounds are easily destroyed through processing, freezing, and some cooking methods, research has investigated the benefits of supplementing with plant sterols and sterolins. One specific product, Moducare™, uses a proprietary process to preserve the ideal combination of sterols and sterolins. More than two decades of clinical research suggest that Moducare™ may be effective in treating a variety of immune-related diseases, such as HIV, pulmonary tuberculosis, stress-induced immune suppression, and even benign prostatic hyperplasia. The plant sterols and sterolins in Moducare™ have anti-inflammatory properties, a fact that may be important in the management of chronic conditions such as rheumatoid arthritis. For more information on these unique plant compounds, look for Lorna Vanderhaeghe's books, *The Immune System Cure* and *Healthy Immunity*.

Oil of Oregano

Oregano is one of the most effective natural antibiotics, with antibacterial, anti-fungal, and antiviral properties. Commonly used to treat infections of the intestines, skin, and lungs, it also acts to strengthen and increase the actions of the immune system.

Studies have found oregano to be an effective treatment against the dangerous bacteria staphylococcus. In one report oregano oil was compared with commonly used drugs (such as penicillin) and determined to be just as effective.[28]

Conclusion

The immune system fights a constant battle against infections, environmental toxins, cellular decay, and, for some of us, cancer. Whether it is the mucous membrane of the eyes, nose, and mouth or the more sophisticated cell- and antibody-mediated immune responses inside our bodies, it's important to balance and occasionally bolster immunity defenses. As we age, this task becomes more and more important, since our lines of defense become less effective. By eating properly, drinking a lot of water each day, and making some healthy lifestyle shifts, we can ensure that the effectiveness of our immune system lasts a lifetime.

12

FIGHT FAT AND WIN!

There is no doubt that we are getting heavier and heavier. A whopping 56.4 percent of Americans are overweight and 19.8 percent are obese.[1] In Canada, a recent survey revealed that 48 percent of Canadians are overweight and 15 percent are obese.[2] These statistics are surprising when you consider that we spend over $33 billion each year on weight-loss products.[3] The problem is that the fad diets and most weight-loss pills don't work—not in the long term. In fact, reports show that one- to two-thirds of weight lost is usually regained within one year and almost all is regained within five.[4] Take comfort— we have some solid recommendations on how to win the battle of the bulge, lose excess body fat, and maintain a healthy body weight as you age.

What Is a Healthy Weight?

You can use a variety of methods to determine whether you are carrying excess weight to the detriment of your health. The most common and easiest is the body mass index (BMI). The BMI is a mathematical formula that correlates height with body fat. It is expressed as weight in kilograms divided by height in meters squared (BMI = kg/m^2). (Refer to Chapter 4 for an easy way to calculate this figure.)

The World Health Organization recognizes obesity as a BMI greater than 30.[5] But there is also a danger zone—a BMI over 27 is associated with an increased risk of developing health problems.[6] The BMI, however, doesn't always tell a true tale. It can be misleading because it only takes into consideration height and weight, not body composition. For instance, a five-foot-five bodybuilder who has low body fat (15 percent), lots of muscle mass, and weighs 180 pounds would have a BMI of 30, suggesting obesity.

Another way to check your weight status and associated health risks is to apply the waist-to-hip ratio; this reflects the proportion of body fat located around the abdomen. An apple-shaped body (a beer belly or large waist) is linked to health problems like heart disease and cancer. A waist-to-hip ratio greater than 0.95 for men and 0.80 for women is thus associated with increased health risk.[7]

Another method involves checking your percentage of body fat with fat calipers or a bioelectric impedance device. According to this measurement, men with more than 25 percent and women with more than 30 percent body fat are considered obese.[8]

Aging and Weight Gain

It is no myth—as we get older, it's easier to gain weight and harder to take it off. This is particularly true for women, who tend to put on pounds on their hips and thighs, becoming pear shaped. Men gain fat around the midsection—like an apple. There are many reasons why we gain weight as we age. Changes in metabolism, in hormone levels, and in our ability to burn fat (thermogenesis) are just some of the variables. Many people become less active with age, so that even if caloric intake remains constant, weight gain occurs owing to less activity.

Factors Affecting Body Weight

Two of the most important factors in weight management are metabolism and thermogenesis. *Metabolism* is the process whereby your body uses food to create energy. It does this by converting food into ATP (adenosine triphosphate), which is used by the muscle cells to provide energy. Your *metabolic rate* is the rate at which your body turns calories into energy. Food that isn't used immediately for energy gets stored as fat, regardless of whether that food consisted of carbohydrates, fat, or protein.

Thermogenesis is the continual burning of calories (body fat) to produce heat and maintain body temperature. As the metabolic rate increases, more heat is produced and greater amounts of fat are burned. A special type of fat cell, known as *brown adipose tissue* (BAT), plays a critical role in the burning of body fat (white fat). In his best-selling book, *Fat Wars*, performance nutritionist Brad King describes the key function of BAT cells in weight control. When you consume a meal, calories are used for energy, stored for future use, or burned by BAT cells. Thus, BAT cells help the body burn excess calories and prevent fat storage. According to King, "It is theorized that the sudden weight gain experienced by many between the ages of 30 to 40 may be the result of a shutdown of the BAT cell thermogenic mechanisms."[9] To prevent the ensuing fat gain, you need to find ways to stimulate BAT cells to break down stored fat.

Understanding Weight Gain

In the past, the first law of thermodynamics was often used to explain what controls body weight. Simply, when energy intake (food) exceeds energy expenditures (exercise/activity), weight gain occurs. It was thus believed that reducing intake and increasing expenditures was the key to weight loss. For years, doctors and researchers believed this simple theory. We now know that other factors are involved. Some people can exercise religiously, reduce food intake, and still not lose weight. And, of course, we all know people who can eat whatever they want and never gain a pound. Weight gain and obesity are complex conditions, dependent upon various lifestyle, hormonal, biochemical, metabolic, and genetic factors. The following are some of the most important factors:

- *Caloric intake.* Overeating and consuming more calories than your body uses for energy can result in weight gain.
- *Quality of food.* Eating too much saturated fat, sugar, processed food, and fast food is associated with weight gain.
- *Stress.* Exposure to chronic stress can cause weight gain, particularly around the midsection. This occurs because stress increases the production and release of cortisol, which increases body fat.
- *Thyroid function.* A sluggish and poorly functioning thyroid can reduce metabolic rate and cause weight gain.
- *Insulin.* When insulin levels are high, the body stores more fat and is unable to use fat as a source of energy.
- *Estrogen.* High levels are associated with weight gain. Why then, you'll likely ask, do women gain weight when their estrogen levels decline in menopause? As a compensatory mechanism, fat cells take on the role of producing estrogen, and to meet the escalating demand, they increase in size and number.
- *Testosterone.* Since testosterone helps the body maintain lean muscle mass and burn fat, a deficiency can lead to loss of muscle mass and fat gain, especially in men.
- *Human growth hormone.* By increasing lean muscle mass and reducing the storage of body fat, human growth hormone regulates body weight. Levels decline with age, particularly after 50, causing a shift in body composition.
- *Genetics.* It has been estimated that genes play a role in 25 percent of the cases of obesity. While you might have an increased risk of obesity because of your genetic background, dietary and environmental factors can affect the expression of these genes.
- *Serotonin.* Because serotonin is the chemical messenger in the brain that regulates satiety, when its levels are low, we feel hungry and when they are higher, we feel satisfied.
- *Leptin.* Satiety is also regulated by leptin, a hormone produced by body fat. Some people become resistant to their own leptin; to compensate for this, the body

produces more and more of the hormone, but the "satisfied" message is not properly received by the brain.

- *Physical activity.* This is one of the most effective ways to boost your metabolism and burn calories. As you exercise, your muscles utilize calories for energy and generate heat, which promotes the burning of fat. Conversely, a lack of exercise causes loss of muscle mass, a reduced metabolic rate, and increased body fat.

Forget the Fads

There is no shortage of weight-loss plans on the market. The barrage of diets, pills, and potions can be very confusing. Be warned: stay away from fads—they just don't work in the long run, and some can be dangerous to your health. As for the weight-loss pills, less than half of those on the market actually work. Most are based on hype rather than science, and few are clinically tested. In the section on supplements below, we will highlight products that have been clinically shown to help with weight loss, but first we will outline dietary strategies that are easy to follow and good for your health.

Losing Body Fat the Healthy Way

To lose excess body fat effectively, you need to use methods that will burn stored body fat and prevent the storage of excess calories as fat. You can do this by activating your BAT and improving metabolism and thermogenesis. By following some simple guidelines for nutrition and exercise and learning about the top weight-loss supplements, you can be well on your way to a trimmer waistline and thinner thighs.

Fat-Burning Diet

In Chapter 7, we provided guidelines for healthy eating and longevity. These principles (eat a balanced diet, choose quality foods, control quantities) can be applied to weight loss as well. However, a few additional suggestions can also help to boost metabolism, curb cravings for sweets, and shed that extra fat.

You can start by modifying the balance of your macronutrient intake in order to achieve a 40-30-30 ratio (carbohydrates-protein-fat). Many health researchers (including Dr. Barry Sears, author of *The Zone*) believe that this is the optimal ratio for reducing body fat. These values differ slightly from the recommendations in Chapter 7; protein intake is higher to reflect the muscles' increased need during weight training, and carbohydrates are reduced to 40 percent because excess carbohydrate consumption can raise insulin levels and be a factor in weight gain.

Pick lean protein sources such as fish, chicken, turkey, eggs, and beans. Red meat is okay in moderation, but it does contain saturated fat and extra calories. Choose carbohydrates with a low glycemic index (see Chapter 19). This will help prevent peaks in blood sugar and insulin (and the resulting fat storage), thwart cravings for sweets, and improve your emotional state.

Increase your intake of the health-promoting essential fatty acids (fish, flaxseed, olive oil), and cut back on saturated fats and trans fats (refer back to Chapter 7).

Don't starve yourself or skip meals. Believe it or not, this can slow your metabolism, lead to loss of muscle mass, and cause your body to hold on to more fat.

Eat small, frequent meals to keep your energy level high, maintain blood-sugar levels, and prevent cravings between meals and overeating at mealtime. Forget the three "squares" and aim for five to six small meals (300–500 calories each).

Don't overeat. Depending on your size and activity level, caloric intake should range between 1,200 and 2,200 calories a day. Eat slowly so that the brain gets the message when you are full. Try to chew each bite of food 10–20 times; this improves digestion and prevents overeating.

Don't drink too much water while eating, but drink plenty of it (6–8 glasses) at other times.

Choose healthy snacks—fruit, vegetables, nuts, seeds, and yogurt. Don't buy junk food; it would just tempt you if it were in the cupboard.

Fat-Fighting Foods

Soy   Soy foods have been shown to improve fat metabolism.[10] Soy is a *phytoestrogen* (plant-based estrogen-like substance) that binds to estrogen receptors in the body, reducing the amount of fat that enters the fat cells.

Flaxseed   Flaxseed is a rich source of *lignans*, which help to balance hormone levels. Body fat contains an enzyme called *aromatase* that converts testosterone into estrogen, high levels of which, as noted, are a factor in weight gain. Lignans have been shown to inhibit aromatase.[11] By preventing this conversion, they may play a role in controlling hormone-related weight gain. Flaxseed is also high in fiber and omega-3 fatty acids.

Fiber   Fiber regulates blood-sugar and insulin levels, improves digestion and elimination, and makes us feel more full with meals (preventing overeating).

Foods to Avoid

- Processed food: refined grains and foods lacking nutritional value and containing added chemicals and preservatives
- Fast food: hamburgers, french fries, and hot dogs, all loaded with saturated fat and calories
- Snack food: chips, pretzels, candy, and soda pop—again, foods high in fat and sugar

Exercises for a Lean Body

Contrary to popular belief, aerobic (cardiovascular) activity on its own does not offer the most effective way to lose body fat. As we learned in Chapter 6, aerobic activities (walking, biking, dancing) do burn calories and provide health benefits (improving heart and lung function, for example), but if your body doesn't have the right fuel available, these activities can also burn muscle—and this goes against what you are trying to accomplish. To boost your metabolism, improve thermogenesis, and lose body fat, you must also do resistance training, such as lifting weights. These exercises build lean muscle mass, and the more muscle you have the more calories you burn. In fact, one pound of muscle burns more than 50 calories a day. Ladies, don't worry about building big, bulky muscles; without hormonal enhancement, it just won't happen.

We're not advising you to cast aside cardiovascular exercise—it is an important element of your workout—but to maximize fat loss, you should undertake a balance of activities, and in a particular order. It was once thought that cardiovascular exercises should be done first, to allow the muscles to warm up and to maximize fat loss. However, during the first 20 minutes of a workout, sugar (carbohydrates), not fat, is the primary source of fuel. So, in order to burn fat calories with aerobic activities at the beginning of your session, you have to do them for more than 20 minutes. Most people don't have time to spend more than 20 minutes on the treadmill or bike. Many sports researchers feel that it's much better to do cardio after your weight-training routine. That way, your body will be switched into fat-burning mode when you start your aerobics, and you can take advantage of the endorphins and hormones (testosterone and growth hormone) that are released after your weight workout.

Here are our recommended resistance and cardiovascular exercises to enhance fat loss and improve body composition.

Resistance Training

Goal Work out with weights for 20–40 minutes every other day.

Exercises Choose two body parts per workout: for example, chest and triceps on Monday, back and biceps on Wednesday, and legs and shoulders on Friday. Vary your exercise routine to challenge your muscles. Pick two exercises per body part and do two to three sets of that move. For example, do chest presses and dumbbell flies to work the chest. Start off by using a lower weight and doing 15–20 repetitions of each move. Over a period of several weeks, increase the weight and lower the repetitions so that you're using a weight that fatigues your muscle in 10–12 repetitions.

Tips Take the time to do the move properly. Bad technique can lead to injury and a less effective workout. Be consistent—don't miss a workout. Find a partner, for motivation and consistency. Seek the advice of a personal trainer to learn how to use the weights and machines properly. Refer to suggestions in Chapter 6 on types of exercises and safety precautions.

Cardiovascular Activity

Goal   Work out for 30 minutes five times per week.

Exercises   Cardiovascular activities include walking, swimming, biking, aerobics, dancing, and rollerblading. Start slowly and gradually increase the duration and intensity of your activities. If you can only do five minutes to start with, that's fine. With time, endurance improves. Pick activities that you enjoy and try to do them first thing in the morning or right after work. To increase intensity, add power to the movements. For example, once you can handle a brisk 30-minute walk with ease, add hand/ankle weights or travel on an incline. For best results, stay with the program and be consistent. Chart your progress and establish rewards for goals you've achieved (not food!).

Tips   The best time to work out is early in the morning or as early in the day as possible; we have more energy then and will continue to burn calories for several hours afterward. Exercise on an empty stomach or after a light snack or shake. If your exercises can't be fit in before work, then try to do them after work. Before a weight routine, warm up with a walk or bike for 5–10 minutes. After the workout, remember to stretch. This will help prevent soreness and fatigue the next day, and it's a great way to relax and cool down.

Cellulite Solution

Even with proper diet and exercise, many people, especially women, have a hard time getting rid of cellulite. In fact, more than 90 percent of women have cellulite. Cellulite is superficial fat that results from impaired circulation and enlargement of fat cells. The connective tissue pulls on the skin, causing the fat cells to glob together; this gives the skin an "orange peel" look. Don't waste your money on expensive creams and potions. None of them have been found to work. The massage technique known as *endermologie* is a helpful way to minimize cellulite. Using suction and rollers, this massage increases circulation, improves fluid exchange, and smoothes the skin's surface. It has been popular in Europe for many years and is now available in North America.

Recommended Supplements

While there is no magic pill for weight loss, some supplements can support this process by enhancing metabolism and thermogenesis, improving energy, and protecting the body against free-radical damage. It's important not to rely solely on these products, but you can make them part of your weight-loss plan.

Antioxidants

Throughout this book, we've emphasized the benefits of antioxidants in combating many age-related diseases. When it comes to weight loss, antioxidants are again an essential part of your program. They protect body cells against free-radical damage, which is accelerated by exercise (and many other body processes). They also support the body during fat loss. Look for an antioxidant blend that contains vitamins C and E, selenium, grape seed extract, coenzyme Q10, and lipoic acid.

Although lipoic acid has not been studied for weight loss, many researchers feel that it offers some benefits through regulation of blood-sugar levels. It improves glucose utilization and reduces the formation of harmful advanced glycation end-products (AGE). These complexes, formed when blood-sugar levels are high, damage cellular proteins and are associated with many age-related diseases. Lipoic acid is thus extremely important as an anti-aging nutrient, since it can reduce the formation of AGE. It is found along with other important anti-aging nutrients in the formula called AGE Inhibitors, by Greens+ Canada.

Citrus Aurantium

Obtained from the bitter Seville orange, citrus aurantium stimulates the release of chemicals in the body that increase metabolic rate and enhance the breakdown of fat. Unlike ephedrine, which has negative effects on the heart and nervous system, citrus aurantium is much better tolerated. Further, it does not cross into the brain or cause anxiety, nervousness, and insomnia, as does ephedrine. Preliminary studies have shown that citrus aurantium supports weight loss.[12] The recommended dose of citrus aurantium is 975–1,200 milligrams per day. It is one of the main ingredients in Trim Fit™ by Quest Vitamins.

Conjugated Linoleic Acid (CLA)

CLA is a derivative of linoleic acid, which is found in foods such as meat and dairy products. It offers a number of health benefits, including protection against cancer and atherosclerosis. As a weight-loss aid, CLA improves fat metabolism and insulin sensitivity.[13] Foods provide only a small amount of CLA—6.1 milligrams per gram of fat in butter and 4.3 milligrams per gram of fat in ground beef. Research with regard to weight loss has found a positive effect at doses of 3–5 grams per day.

Chromium

Chromium is an essential trace mineral that has some similar properties to lipoic acid. It works with insulin to move glucose into cells and thus is an important nutrient for blood-sugar control. At doses of 400 micrograms per day, it promotes weight loss, reducing body fat and improving lean muscle mass.[14]

Green Tea

Gaining in popularity as a health drink, green tea offers a number of health benefits; for example, it reduces risk factors for heart disease and offers protection against cancer. Green tea is rich in catechins, a type of antioxidant. It also contains caffeine (about 50 milligrams per cup). Some preliminary research suggests that the combination of these ingredients promotes weight loss by increasing energy expenditures (burning calories).[15] Green tea is often used in combination with other thermogenic ingredients, such as citrus aurantium.

Phase 2™

Phase 2™, a standardized extract derived from the white kidney bean, promotes weight loss by blocking the digestion of dietary starch. It works in the intestine by inhibiting the activity of alpha amylase, the enzyme that converts starch into smaller glucose molecules for absorption. Over-consumption of starches is a factor in weight gain. Phase 2™ works to neutralize some of those starch calories. It has been shown to reduce blood sugar after starchy meals and promote loss of body fat.[16] Since the product acts in the intestine and is not absorbed into the bloodstream, it is very well tolerated and not likely to interact with other drugs or supplements. The recommended dose of Phase 2™ is 500–1,000 milligrams once or twice daily before meals.

Whey Protein

Certain types of whey protein stimulate the hormone cholecystokinin (CCK), which controls feelings of hunger. CCK sends satiety signals to the brain, thus helping to prevent overeating. CCK has other important functions: for example, it improves gallbladder function and bowel motility.[17] Very few whey proteins have the ability to stimulate CCK production. Look for AlphaPure™ brand. This special whey protein is also found in AGE Inhibitors, mentioned above.

Conclusion

There is no quick and easy route to safe and effective weight loss. For long-term success, you need to emphasize healthy eating and physical activity—and this takes work and motivation. You've heard these words before and they're true—you didn't put the weight on overnight, and you're not going to take it off overnight. Set realistic goals and be patient with yourself. Health authorities agree that slow, gradual weight loss (one to two pounds per week) is a safe goal. Supplements can play a role in weight loss, but they should not become a crutch. Seek advice from your health-care professional so that you can develop a personalized plan to help you realize your goals.

13

OSTEOPOROSIS: OUTWITTING THE SILENT THIEF

Like a thief who, unknown to you, steals a coin every day for years on end, osteoporosis can rob you of your bone health bit by bit for many years without presenting any symptoms. Referred to as the "silent thief," osteoporosis (which means "porous bones") is a disease that thins and weakens bones to the point where they can easily fracture, usually in the hip, spine, or wrist. The risk of osteoporosis increases with age, but age is not the only risk factor. In this chapter, we will explore what you can do to prevent osteoporosis, stop bone loss, and even build bone.

The Growing Epidemic

Osteoporosis afflicts more than 25 million Americans, leading to 1.5 million bone fractures a year and an estimated $14 billion in treatment costs. One in three women over 50 will suffer a vertebral fracture.[1] The picture is similar in Canada: 1.4 million Canadians suffer from the disease, with an estimated annual health bill of $1.3 billion.[2] As the number of older adults in our society continues to increase, so do these figures.

Bone Basics

Bone consists of a matrix of protein fibers (collagen) hardened with calcium, phosphorus, magnesium, zinc, copper, and other minerals. An interconnecting structure gives bone its strength. On the outside, there's a tough, dense rind of bone; on the inside, spongy-looking bone.

Bone is living tissue and is thus in a constant state of growth and deterioration. Special cells called *osteoclasts* are constantly breaking down old bone matter, and at the same time, cells called *osteoblasts* are replacing it with new tissue. The activity of these cells is regulated primarily by hormones—estrogen, testosterone, and parathyroid hormone. As people age, more bone is broken down than is replaced. The inside of a bone normally looks like a honeycomb, but when osteoporosis is present, the spaces in that honeycomb grow larger, as more bone is destroyed than replaced. This makes bones weaker and more susceptible to fracture.

Before a person reaches 30, there's a relative balance between the work of osteoclasts and osteoblasts. After that point, bone loss begins, albeit at a very slow rate. In women, the rate of loss accelerates for several years after menopause, then slows again. But osteoporosis is not just a woman's disease. With age, men also experience changes in hormone levels that put them at risk, but these changes occur more slowly and at a later stage in life. By the time they reach their sixties, men and women lose bone at about the same rate. The key is to build strong healthy bones early in life in order to be in a better position in later years.

It's not fully understood why osteoporosis occurs, but a number of risk factors have been identified. Some of these factors we have control over (modifiable risk factors); others we cannot change (unmodifiable risk factors). Modifiable risk factors include the following:

- Poor diet (low calcium and vitamin D consumption; high intake of sodium, animal protein, and caffeine)
- Inactivity (being a couch potato)
- Smoking
- Anorexia
- Excessive alcohol consumption (more than three drinks a day)
- Low hormone levels (estrogen in women, testosterone in men)
- Use of certain medications (cortisone and anticonvulsants)

These are some of the unmodifiable risk factors:

- Age (risk increases with age, particularly over age 50)
- Gender (women are more susceptible than men)
- Ethnicity (Caucasian and Asian women are more susceptible)
- Body frame (those with small, thin bones are more likely to be affected)
- Family history

Symptoms and Diagnosis

Most people don't realize they have osteoporosis until a sudden strain, bump, or fall causes a hip to fracture or a vertebra to collapse. Collapsed vertebrae may initially be felt or seen in the form of severe back pain, loss of height, or spinal deformities such as kyphosis (severely stooped posture).

Bone mineral density (BMD) is a term used to describe the solidity of bones. The most accurate way to measure bone density is with a DEXA-scan (dual-energy X-ray absorptiometry), a painless, non-invasive, safe, and accurate method. Since DEXA-scans are costly, they are usually only used with women over 50 and people with risk factors for osteoporosis. The DEXA-scan is used to determine bone density, confirm a diagnosis, predict risk of fracture, and monitor the effects of treatment (if any). The results are reported as a number that tells you how your bone density measures up against that of a healthy adult without osteoporosis. For example, a result of –2.5 SD (standard deviation) or greater indicates the presence of osteoporosis. A test result between –1 SD and –2.5 SD means there is some bone loss (a condition known as osteopenia) and some risk of osteoporosis. If tests are done at least a year apart, doctors can compare the results and determine whether treatment is slowing the bone loss.

Prevention

While some degree of bone loss occurs with age, that is no reason to be complacent. Just as we contribute to retirement plans in order to be financially stable in later life, we can contribute to our bone mineral density early on to prevent osteoporosis and ensure the best possible bone health as we age. Furthermore, the financial advice that it's never too late to start saving for retirement applies to bone health as well. There are many things we can do throughout our lives to improve the health of our bones.

Exercise

Exercise is an important component of any osteoporosis prevention and treatment program. Weight-bearing activities, those that place stress on the bone, strengthen bones and improve bone density. Though weight training is an obvious example of weight-bearing exercise, walking, playing tennis, jogging, and aerobics also force you to work against gravity.

Older adults benefit from weight-training or weight-bearing exercise. Physical fitness reduces the risk of fractures due to falls through improved balance, muscle strength, and agility. Studies have shown that exercise during adulthood can reduce falls by approximately 25 percent.[3]

So how much exercise do your bones need? Most authorities recommend 30 minutes of weight-bearing activity five times a week. Chapter 6 offered some guidelines about how to get started. While exercise is good for people with osteoporosis, they should consult with a physician and personal trainer before undertaking an exercise program. It's especially important that they take care to avoid injury.

Nutrition

Proper nutrition is essential for healthy bodies and healthy bones. When it comes to bone health, we need to pay particular attention to calcium, vitamin D, and soy foods.

Calcium

Adequate calcium consumption is critical for the prevention and treatment of osteoporosis. Low calcium levels are associated with low bone mass, rapid bone loss, and high fracture rates.[4] Although adequate amounts of calcium can be obtained through a healthy diet, recent studies have shown that we are not getting enough. Many people consume less than half the recommended daily amount of calcium necessary to build and maintain healthy bones. This is especially true among girls and young women, those who need it most.[5]

Healthy calcium-rich foods include low-fat dairy foods (cheese, yogurt, milk); canned fish with bones you can eat (salmon, sardines); dark-green leafy vegetables (kale, collards, broccoli); calcium-fortified orange juice; and breads made with calcium-fortified flour.

Three to four servings of dairy products each day provide about 1,200 milligrams of calcium. A serving is the equivalent of 1 cup of milk, pudding, or yogurt; 1 ounce of cheese; or 2 cups of cottage cheese. Try to use low- or non-fat foods whenever possible.

The recommended daily requirement of calcium varies with age. More is needed during childhood and adolescence while bones are rapidly growing, during pregnancy and lactation, and then again after age 50, when hormone levels change, the body is less efficient at absorbing calcium, and there's a greater risk of bone loss. Children under 4 years of age should have 500 milligrams of calcium per day. From ages 4 to 8, the daily recommended calcium intake increases to 800 milligrams; from ages 9 to 18, it increases to 1,300 milligrams per day. From 19 to 50, the recommended daily intake drops to 1,000 milligrams, only to increase to 1,200 milligrams per day after age 51.[6]

If your calcium intake falls short of the recommended daily amounts, you should consider taking a calcium supplement. There are many different forms of calcium to choose from: carbonate, citrate, lactate, chelate, and others. Carbonate, the least expensive of these forms, provides the highest amount of elemental calcium but can cause constipation and gas. As well, people over age 50 and/or with low stomach acid may have problems absorbing it into their systems. The citrates and chelates are well absorbed, affordable, and more easily tolerated.

Calcium supplements are very safe when taken at recommended doses. As much as 2,500 milligrams can be safely taken by most people on a daily basis.[7] Doses above this level may be safe for some, but others may experience side effects. If you're at risk of kidney stones, discuss calcium supplements with your doctor before taking them.

Vitamin D

The body needs vitamin D to absorb calcium.[8] In fact, vitamin D can increase calcium absorption by as much as 30–80 percent. Our bodies produce vitamin D when our skin is exposed to sunlight. We also receive it in such foods as fortified milk products and breakfast cereals. Older adults and those who are rarely exposed to sunlight or who are taking medication that impairs vitamin D absorption may require a supplement. The usual supplement dosage is between 400 and 800 IU per day.

Soy Foods

Soy foods such as tofu, soy milk, roasted soy beans, soy powders, and soy bars also play a role in the prevention of osteoporosis.[9] The isoflavones in soy foods are structurally similar to estrogen and produce estrogen-like effects in certain parts of the body, such as bone. Research suggests that there are lower bone fracture rates in cultures that consume large quantities of soy foods.[10] As a result, North American interest in the bone benefits of soy has been increasing over the past decade.

Essential Fatty Acids (EFAs)

Include plenty of EFAs in your diet, as these "good" fats are important elements for maintaining calcium balance and bone mineral density. The omega-3 and omega-6 fatty acids, which are found, respectively in cold-water fish (salmon, herring, mackerel) and the oils of evening primrose, black currant, and borage plants are particularly beneficial.

In a study of older women with osteoporosis, 4 grams of fish oil taken every day for four months resulted in higher blood levels of calcium and better calcium absorption and bone growth.[11] Fish oil combined with evening primrose oil may offer additional benefits. In another study, women received 6 grams of evening primrose oil with fish oil in addition to 600 milligrams of calcium daily for 36 months.[12] Bone deterioration was arrested in the first 18 months, while a group not receiving the treatment lost 3.2 percent of their spinal bone mineral density. During the next 18 months, those women taking evening primrose oil with fish oil had a significant 3.1 percent increase in spinal bone mineral density.

Foods to Avoid

Certain foods, especially junk foods, have a negative effect on bone health. Too much caffeine (more than three cups of coffee per day) or sodium can increase the loss of calcium through urination, accelerating bone deterioration.[13] Naturally, these factors are even more important when you're not receiving the recommended levels of calcium in your diet.

Some research has linked diets high in animal protein to lower bone density and an increased risk of osteoporosis. When dietary protein increases, so does calcium loss through urination.[14] Those who consume the most animal protein (through meat, poultry, and dairy products) have a significantly higher risk of fractures due to osteoporosis than do those who eat the least.[15] Higher protein intake has also been associated with increased hip fractures.[16] It might logically follow that vegetarians would have a lower risk of osteoporosis, but the evidence is inconclusive. To further complicate the issue, since the body needs protein to build bone, a deficiency of protein or a low-protein diet may increase the risk of fracture. Until more is known about the links between vegetarianism and bone health, switching to a vegetarian diet strictly for reasons of bone health cannot be recommended. People who enjoy eating meat should simply do so in moderation.

Soft drinks may also have a negative impact on bone health. Some reports suggest that cola drinkers have an increased incidence of bone fracture and that the risks of fracture seem to increase if you drink large quantities of cola drinks over the long term.[17] The phosphoric acid that's in many soft drinks has been linked to an increased loss of calcium in the urine. In one study, children who consumed at least 1.5 liters per week of soft drinks containing phosphoric acid had more than five times the risk of developing low blood levels of calcium as other children.[18] While these studies may make a strong case, more research is needed. Since these drinks are full of sugar and chemicals and provide no nutritional value, you should minimize your consumption or avoid them altogether.

Supplements That Aid Bone Health

As was indicated earlier, calcium and vitamin D are critical nutrients for bone health. However, the growth and health of our bones require more than a glass of milk and some sunshine. Several other important nutrients are involved in the complex processes of bone development, and some of us may have to rely on nutritional supplements in order to ensure we receive all the necessary elements we need to maintain healthy bones.

Since individual needs and dosages vary, it is important to consult with a qualified health-care practitioner before taking supplements.

Magnesium

Magnesium is a necessary component of bone; in fact, half the body's magnesium stores are found in bone, and many practitioners feel that it plays a valuable role in the treatment and prevention of osteoporosis. Magnesium is required by the enzymes that convert vitamin D into its active form. It is also involved in the secretion of parathyroid hormone and calcitonin, two hormones that regulate bone health.

Several studies have found a correlation between magnesium deficiency and an increased risk of osteoporosis. As well, magnesium blood and bone levels are lower in people with osteoporosis.[19] Magnesium deficiency may be caused by poor diet, alcoholism, or a range of chronic illnesses. Supplemental magnesium reduces bone loss and increases bone mass.[20] For this reason, many doctors recommend that people with osteoporosis supplement their diets with 250–350 milligrams of magnesium each day. Those with a chronic disease or who are at risk of deficiency (poor diet) should also consider a magnesium supplement.

In high doses or when used in certain forms (such as magnesium oxide), magnesium can cause diarrhea. Magnesium citrate and magnesium chelate are the preferred forms, since they are better tolerated. Calcium with magnesium, in a 2:1 ratio, is also less likely to cause an upset stomach.

Silicon and Other Significant Nutrients

Silicon plays a significant role in bone formation, and at least one study has indicated that supplementation with silicon increases bone mineral density in osteoporosis sufferers.[21] While the optimal amount of silicon supplementation remains unknown, some nutritional supplements now contain small amounts.

Boron, copper, manganese, phosphorus, vitamin K, and zinc are other nutrients involved in bone formation. Deficiencies of these substances have been linked to an increased risk of osteoporosis. For this reason, we often find these nutrients in synergistic bone formulas, along with calcium, magnesium, and vitamin D.

Ipriflavone

Ipriflavone, a synthetic isoflavone derived from soy, is used worldwide as a mainstream approach to the treatment and prevention of osteoporosis. It stimulates bone-building activity, inhibits osteoclasts, and reduces bone pain caused by osteoporosis and fractures. When taken in conjunction with calcium, ipriflavone prevents bone loss and reduces the incidence of osteoporotic bone fractures.[22] It has also demonstrated positive effects when used in combination with low doses of estrogen. Iprigen™ is the most widely studied brand of ipriflavone and is available in bone formulas such as Osteo-Logic™ by Quest Vitamins. The recommended dosage is 200 milligrams, taken three times daily with meals.

Drug Therapy

The goal of any treatment for osteoporosis is to stop bone loss and promote bone growth. Proper nutrition and exercise are the cornerstones of this strategy, but some people need the additional help of drug therapy either to slow the rate of bone loss or promote bone development.

Hormone Therapy

Estrogen plays an important role in bone health. In premenopausal women, it slows bone loss through its effect on osteoclasts. When menopause occurs, estrogen levels decline and bone loss accelerates. Doctors often recommend estrogen to post-menopausal women at risk of developing osteoporosis, as it reduces menopausal symptoms and protects against bone loss. Post-menopausal women who have not had a hysterectomy and take estrogen should also take progesterone to protect against uterine cancer. Progesterone, too, has a positive effect on osteoblasts, the bone building cells, and may thus also help prevent osteoporosis.[23]

Not all women will develop osteoporosis as a result of menopause. Nutritional habits, genetics, and lifestyle are other strong determinants. Anyone involved in hormone therapy should recognize the health risks and side effects of these treatments. You should thoroughly discuss all the options with your physician before making any decisions.

Selective Estrogen Receptor Modulators (SERMs)

Raloxifene (Evista®) is a new class of drug approved for the prevention and treatment of osteoporosis. It prevents bone loss and can reduce the incidence of spinal fracture.[24] Unlike estrogen, raloxifene does not increase the risk of cancer of the uterine lining, although it may cause hot flashes and increased risk of blood clots.

Bisphosphonates

Alendronate (Fosamac®), etidronate (Didrocal®), and risedronate (Actonel®) are three drugs that slow bone deterioration and may even increase bone density. They are also effective in battling osteoporosis in men.[25] Side effects can include nausea, heartburn, and pain in the stomach, muscles, and bones.

Calcitonin

Calcitonin (Miacalcin®) is a naturally occurring hormone that controls the activity of bone cells. A synthetic form of this hormone is available as a nasal spray for the prevention and treatment of osteoporosis. Calcitonin slows the osteoclastic deterioration of bones, allowing bone building to overtake the natural rate of bone loss. The result is an increase in bone mass and a reduced risk of fractures. Calcitonin also reduces the pain of fractures. Side effects, which are minimal, include runny or dry nose and skin irritation.

Conclusion

Unless this growing problem is addressed quickly, the incidence of osteoporosis—together with its cost to society—will continue to increase as the North American population grows older. Osteoporosis is preventable, not inevitable. You need to be aware of the modifiable risks associated with osteoporosis and make the necessary lifestyle changes to improve your bone health.

There are straightforward ways to add to your bone-health stores, increasing or at least maintaining your bone mineral density as you prepare for the time in your life when calcium loss becomes inevitable. A diet rich in calcium and vitamin D, regular weight-bearing exercise, and nutritional supplements are key elements in your fight against osteoporosis. If you are diligent about maintaining a bone-healthy lifestyle, you can keep osteoporosis, the silent thief, at bay and avoid being robbed of mobility and independence in later life.

14

SEE ME, HEAR ME

Good eyesight and hearing is something many young adults take for granted. It's not until problems develop that we worry about these vital senses. Unfortunately, some degree of visual loss and hearing impairment is inevitable with aging. A number of interventions, however, slow down these degenerative processes. Lifestyle factors such as diet, exercise, and environment, as well as the use of nutritional supplements, play important roles in protecting our vision and hearing. In this chapter, we will explore some of the most common hearing and vision deficiencies, how they affect us, how we can detect them, and what we can do—and eat—to avoid them or minimize their effect.

Aging and Vision

In Canada, visual impairment affects 9 percent of the population aged 65 and over, or one in 11 seniors.[1] In the United States, more than 11 million people are affected.[2] The leading causes of visual loss are age-related macular degeneration (AMD), cataracts, glaucoma, diabetic retinopathy, optic nerve disease, and eye injuries.

Loss of vision ranks third after arthritis and heart disease as a cause of impaired function in elderly individuals. The economic consequences are staggering: it is estimated that the cost of care and services for the visually impaired exceeds $22 billion each year.[3]

Common Causes of Vision Loss

Age-Related Macular Degeneration

AMD is the leading cause of visual impairment in those age 75 and older.[4] It is caused by damage to the cells in the macula (the back of the retina), the area responsible for providing color and fine detail in the center of our visual field. There are two forms of AMD, dry and wet. The dry form, which accounts for 90 percent of cases, causes a slow and gradual loss of vision over many years. The most common early symptom is progressively worsening blurred central vision. The wet form occurs when new blood vessels behind the retina start to grow towards the macula, causing leakage of fluid and loss of vision. This form is much more severe and threatening to vision. Its noticeable early signs include loss of central vision and the wavy appearance of straight lines.

The exact cause of AMD is unknown, but the risk increases with age, smoking, high cholesterol levels, sunlight exposure, and its presence in family history. Women, Caucasians, and people with blue eyes may also be at greater risk. Those who follow a diet low in antioxidants may also have a greater likelihood of developing AMD.

At present, there is no treatment for dry AMD, but newer laser techniques may be effective with the wet form. Prevention is key: avoid risk factors such as smoking and sunlight exposure, control your cholesterol levels, and consider dietary measures and supplements that offer protection.

Glaucoma

Glaucoma is an eye disease characterized by increased intra-ocular (inside the eyeball) pressure that leads to damage to the optic nerve and blindness. It is the second leading cause of blindness in North America. Although anyone can develop glaucoma, those at particular risk are people over 60, diabetics, blacks, and those with glaucoma in their family history. This is another condition that rarely shows any symptoms in its early stages. As the disease advances, peripheral vision is impaired, creating tunnel vision, and eventually, forward vision diminishes and blindness sets in. Glaucoma cannot be cured, but it can be controlled if detected early enough. Regular eye exams are crucial.

Treatment of glaucoma involves medication that controls the increased eye pressure; it can also involve laser and other surgical procedures. Vitamin C has been used successfully to lower intra-ocular pressure.[5] Some preliminary evidence suggests that alpha lipoic acid and magnesium supplements may be helpful.[6]

Cataracts

Age-related cataracts are a major cause of blindness in Americans, accounting for one out of every seven new cases in people age 45 and older.[7] Cataracts develop when the proteins (crystallins) in the lens of the eye are damaged. This results in clouding of the lens and varying degrees of visual loss. The risk of developing cataracts increases with age, from 10 percent for those under 65 to more than 30 percent for those over 75.[8] Other risk factors include smoking, excessive exposure to sunlight, diabetes, and inflammation.[9]

Neither drugs nor dietary supplements can reverse cataracts; surgical removal is the only treatment. In fact, cataract extraction is one of the most common surgical procedures performed in North America. Prevention is the key to improving quality of life and reducing disability. Researchers estimate that if the progression of cataracts could be delayed by 10 years, the number of cataract surgeries per year would be reduced by 45 percent.[10] By wearing sunglasses, eating fruits and vegetables (rich sources of antioxidants), and avoiding smoking, we can reduce our risk and delay the onset of cataracts.

Diabetic Retinopathy

Diabetic retinopathy is a common complication of diabetes. It occurs when the retinal blood vessels break down and leak fluid, causing visual loss or blindness. All diabetics are at risk, and almost half will develop some degree of this disease during their lifetime. There is no pain, and symptoms often don't develop until the disease becomes severe. This is why regular eye exams are so important; diabetics should go at least once a year.

Treatment of diabetic retinopathy involves laser surgery to seal the leaking blood vessels. While it does not restore vision, it significantly reduces the risk of severe vision loss. Keeping tight control of blood-sugar levels is the best way to slow the onset and progression of diabetic retinopathy.

Nutrients and Eye Health

A number of nutrients and herbs can aid your vision. The products discussed below have been clinically studied and shown to be beneficial for the prevention and treatment of eye disease.

The Carotenoids

If your mother told you to eat carrots because they are good for your eyes, she was right! Carrots are a rich source of beta carotene, the precursor to vitamin A and essential for eye health. It has long been known that a vitamin A deficiency can cause night blindness. A lack of zinc can also be a factor, since vitamin A requires zinc to work properly. Supplementing with vitamin A and zinc is thus helpful in correcting night blindness in those with deficiencies.

Carotenoids are highly colored (red, orange, yellow) plant pigments possessing significant antioxidant activity. Other nutrients in the carotenoid family that play a strong role in vision are lutein and zeaxanthin, pigments found in many leafy green and yellow vegetables. These pigments are the only carotenoids present in the macular pigment of the eye. It is believed that they function as antioxidants to protect the eye against free-radical damage and to absorb damaging ultraviolet light. Research has shown that a significantly lower risk of AMD is associated with both higher blood levels of lutein and zeaxanthin and high dietary intake of foods rich in these pigments (kale, collard greens, spinach, and broccoli).[11]

Lutein and zeaxanthin are also found in the human lens, and preliminary research has found that they lower the risk of cataracts.[12] While a deficiency of beta carotene is rare in our society, we could improve our intake of lutein and zeaxanthin. Research suggests an average intake of only 0.57 milligrams per day,[13] much less than the 6 milligrams recommended for prevention.

Bilberry

Bilberry contains antioxidant chemicals called *anthocyanosides* that speed the regeneration of the purple pigment in the eye used for night vision.[14] For this reason, bilberry is used to treat night blindness.[15] Anthocyanosides also support the normal formation of connective tissue, strengthen capillaries in the body, and may improve blood flow. Bilberry may be helpful in the prevention of cataracts and the treatment of AMD and diabetic retinopathy. The usual dose for bilberry is 240–600 milligrams per day of a product standardized to provide 25 percent anthocyanosides. There are no known side effects or drug interactions with bilberry.

Antioxidants

The antioxidants vitamins C and E and glutathione offer a variety of benefits for eye health. Vitamin C is needed to activate vitamin E, which in turn activates glutathione. Supplementing your diet with vitamins C and E can lower the risk of cataracts and possibly AMD.[16] Moreover, vitamin C supplements can significantly reduce elevated intra-ocular pressure in individuals with glaucoma.[17] The recommended intake for vitamin C varies with age and nutritional status. Smokers need extra vitamin C, as do those under stress or taking certain prescription drugs. Supplemental doses may range between 200 and 2,000 milligrams per day. Higher doses (greater than 2 grams) appear to offer greater benefits for lowering intra-ocular pressure in those with glaucoma.

Vitamin E prevents blood from clotting too fast and protects diabetics' blood vessels from damage.[18] Animal studies have shown that vitamin E protects against cataracts.[19] Most studies found benefits with doses between 50 and 800 IU.

Ginkgo Biloba

Ginkgo biloba, one of the most widely researched plants, offers a range of health benefits. As an antioxidant, it offers protection against free-radical damage associated with many age-related diseases. Ginkgo exerts its effects in the brain, retina, and cardiovascular system.[20] It may help in the treatment of early-stage macular degeneration,[21] and it has been found to improve diabetic retinopathy.[22] The usual recommended dose is 120–240 milligrams of a standardized extract, such as Ginkoba™ by Pharmaton.

Hearing Loss

We've all watched comical scenes in movies and cartoons featuring elderly folk who misunderstand everything being said around them. It is an exaggerated image but one that bears some truth. There is indeed a direct link between aging and hearing loss. You should take great care to reduce your risks of hearing loss and recognize when you have a problem.

Hearing loss is a common condition in the Western world's older population. People over 65 constituted 12.8 percent of the American population in 1995, but they accounted for about 37 percent of those who reported hearing impairments.[23] Likely, the latter number would be even higher if all instances of hearing loss were reported. The incidence of hearing impairment has been increasing for years. Between 1971 and 1991 the number of people who experienced hearing impairment in the United States jumped 53.4 percent, moving from 69 per 1,000 to slightly more than 86 per 1,000.[24] As the baby boomer generation graduates into old age, these numbers will rise even more.

The causes of hearing loss are varied. Genetics, persistent ear infections, disease, injury, medication, vitamin deficiencies, and smoking all play a role, but the two most common causes of hearing loss are *presbycusis* (the gradual loss of hearing that occurs with aging) and noise-induced impairment. Presbycusis is a natural process believed to involve the gradual stiffening of the hairs of the inner ear. Noise-induced hearing loss, however, is not a natural process but is becoming more common as the first generation to grow up with loud rock music settles into middle and later life.

Former punk rock guitarist Kathy Peck knows well the effects of noise-induced hearing loss. She experienced hearing loss after performing a concert in 1984; four years later she co-founded Hearing Education and Awareness for Rockers (HEAR) with California medical doctor Flash Gordon. HEAR acts as an information and resource service, working with high-profile rock musicians to promote its cause via radio, television, the Internet, and music events throughout the United States.[25]

Tinnitus

After that fateful 1984 concert, one symptom of Peck's hearing loss was a ringing sensation in her ears. Though usually a temporary condition for concert-goers, ringing or buzzing in the ears—called tinnitus—is a chronic condition for an estimated 40–50 million Americans,[26] often affecting their quality of life. Their sleep is disturbed, their concentration at work is disrupted, and in some cases the frustration and stress of the condition leads to mental health problems. Tinnitus is also associated with hyperacusis, a hearing condition that increases sensitivity to moderate-to-loud noises.

Tinnitus is generally caused by the cumulative effects of loud noise, whether at a concert, in the workplace, or during recreational activities like those involving firearms or motorized vehicles. It is also caused by age-related changes in the inner ear, explaining the higher incidence of this condition in older people. Other possible contributing factors include severe blows to the head, impacted ear wax, a dysfunctional joint in the jaw bone, stress, Ménière's disease, some types of prescription medication, and large doses of Aspirin and certain other drugs.[27]

Sufferers can often control tinnitus by keeping a regular sleep schedule, exercising daily, cutting down on caffeine, alcohol, and salt, reducing stress, and avoiding loud noise. Some prescription medications provide relief for those who are debilitated by the condition. Alternatively, some have found relief using melatonin, ginkgo biloba, and vitamin B12 injections. Melatonin is a hormone in the brain that helps regulate sleep, but it is also produced synthetically and, in regulated doses, can help tinnitus sufferers better cope with their condition.[28] Ginkgo biloba, a herbal extract produced from the leaves of ancient Chinese ginkgo trees, increases blood circulation[29] and thereby helps the cells of the body, including those of the inner ear, get more oxygen. Vitamin B12, important for proper nerve functioning,[30] can enhance the health of the hearing nerves in the ears.

Maskers, devices that create an overriding sound that is less troubling to hear, can also be used to reduce the effects of tinnitus. They are available in several forms, ranging from a table-top device, to one that is inserted in the ear, to another that is used in combination with hearing aids.[31]

Prevention

While we have some control over the causes of noise-induced hearing loss, there is little we can do to prevent age-related hearing loss. We can, however, delay its onset by maintaining the healthy hearing practices listed here:

- Reduce exposure to loud noises. Any noise at 85 decibels or more can contribute to hearing loss over time. Listening to loud music with headphones can be harmful to your hearing. Wear earplugs when you know you'll be exposed to loud noises for long periods of time.
- Quit smoking. A 1998 study suggests that smokers are 1.69 times more likely to experience hearing loss.[32]
- Try to avoid contracting ear infections. Repeated ear infections can cause lasting damage to the fragile components of the ear.
- Avoid exposing your ears to extreme weather conditions, such as cold and wind.
- Exercise regularly. Regular exercise helps you maintain healthy circulation throughout your body.

- Avoid extended exposure to chemicals that can damage hearing. If you handle chemicals at work or at home, it is important to know what you're working with and what effects it can have on you.
- Have regular hearing tests. You should have your hearing tested every couple of years. Hearing loss is a very gradual process, one that you wouldn't readily notice without the help of an audiologist or other hearing specialist.

Hearing Aids

If hearing impairment is properly identified and addressed, hearing aids allow people to continue enjoying the voices and other sounds around them. Several types of hearing aids are available, ranging in price, size, quality, and complexity. In the past, hearing aids carried a stigma of old age. This image is changing, though, with some prominent younger people now wearing them. Former American president Bill Clinton, for example, was only 51 when during his second term in office he was fitted with digital hearing aids.

You should banish from your mind any preconceived images you might have of hearing-aid wearers. It's far better to enjoy the benefits of improved hearing than to worry about some imagined stigma.

Conclusion

There are a number of ways to preserve your vision and hearing with age, the most important of which involve lifestyle choices. Smoking increases the risk of eye disease and hearing loss—another reason to quit. Regular exercise improves circulation and blood flow throughout the body. A diet rich in fruits and vegetables provides the antioxidants that protect the eyes. Supplements of the carotenoids, bilberry, and the other nutrients discussed are highly recommended for those at risk of AMD and cataracts. Tight control of blood-sugar levels is crucial for diabetics and those at risk of retinopathy. Loud noise is to be avoided as much as possible—it's not rude to wear earplugs, unless you are tuning out your spouse. Lastly, it is important to have regular vision and hearing exams. The earlier that problems are identified and treated, the better your chances of preserving these vital senses.

15

WOMEN'S HEALTH: MENOPAUSE AND BEYOND

In a woman's lifetime, her body goes through many changes in response to the natural rise and fall of hormones. In the reproductive years, from puberty to menopause, cyclical hormonal variations prepare women for child bearing. In menopause, hormone levels wane. While many women have anxiety about this phase, it is actually a time to be embraced. There are many options when it comes to managing menopausal symptoms, and it is truly possible for women to enjoy health and vitality during these years.

Ovarian Retirement

Menopause is not a disease or illness. It is a natural phase in a woman's life, occurring naturally between the ages of 40 and 55. During menopause, ovulation ceases and women lose their ability to conceive children. The ovaries have gone into retirement. The menstrual cycle may end suddenly, or it may taper off gradually over a period of years, a phase known as *perimenopause*, the years before menopause. When one year has passed without a menstrual period, a woman is considered to be in menopause.

The Symptoms

The symptoms of menopause are caused by the decline in hormone levels as the ovaries shut down. The hormones most affected are estrogen, progesterone, and sometimes testosterone. Some women experience few if any symptoms, while others have a very difficult time. If the hormones decline gradually, the body can more easily adapt to the changing levels and symptoms might be less severe. Women who exercise regularly, eat a healthy diet, abstain from caffeine, sugar, and alcohol, and practice stress management also have an easier time. The most common symptoms of menopause are hot flashes, mood swings, irritability, vaginal and skin dryness, night sweats, and insomnia.

Hot Flashes

Hot flashes, the focus of many menopause jokes, are no laughing matter for anyone experiencing them. They begin suddenly on the chest, neck, and face, causing increased warmth, sweating, and reddening of the skin. They can last between three and six minutes and occur several times a day. Hot flashes interfere with sleep and concentration, and cause headaches, nausea, dizziness, and fatigue.

Vaginal Symptoms

Estrogen keeps the vaginal tissue strong, elastic, and lubricated. During menopause, reduced estrogen levels lead to dryness and thinning of the vagina. Over time, the vagina actually shrinks in size, becoming narrower and shorter. All of these symptoms can make intercourse uncomfortable and even painful.

Emotional Symptoms

Some women have emotional problems—mood swings, irritability, anxiety, depression, and crying spells. These symptoms are similar to those of premenstrual syndrome (PMS), and both sets of symptoms seem to be related to fluctuating estrogen levels. Although some women feel depressed during menopause, true clinical depression is not a direct consequence of the low estrogen levels of menopause. Many women see menopause as an end of their youth, sexuality, and beauty. These feelings may be compounded by the way society associates beauty with youth. Negative perceptions about menopause, lack of spousal support, and poor marital relations can also contribute to a woman's depression.

Sexuality and Menopause

While a woman's reproductive ability is lost with menopause, her sexuality remains. Nevertheless, certain physical and psychological changes can affect a woman's sex life. The pain or discomfort during intercourse caused by vaginal dryness and thinning may reduce her interest in sexual activity. As well, sexual desire or libido may diminish as hormone levels decrease. Even so, women are still capable of having intimate sexual relations well beyond the menopausal years.

Bladder Blues

Recurrent bladder infections affect about 15 percent of menopausal women.[1] Symptoms include burning pain during urination, urinary frequency and urgency, and clouding of the urine. Some women experience urinary incontinence, typically after sneezing, coughing, laughing, or lifting a heavy object. These symptoms are the result of estrogen deprivation in the muscle and tissues around the vagina and bladder. Weak pelvic muscles can be a contributing factor.

Kegel exercises can prevent or reduce the degree of incontinence by strengthening the pubococcygeus (PC) muscle—the band of muscle that circles the vagina. A tighter PC muscle can reduce urinary incontinence and improve sexual pleasure. If you are not sure where this muscle is, the next time you are urinating, try to stop the flow of urine. The inner pelvic muscle that you contract to do this is your PC muscle. Practice this several times a day when you urinate; try to hold the urine back for five seconds at a time and then gradually increase the length of time. Another way to find this muscle is to insert two fingers into your vagina. Separate those fingers and try to use your pubic muscle to push them back together. After you become acquainted with this muscle, you can do these exercises lying on the floor, sitting in the car, or standing in line at the bank. It may take a month or so to notice the difference. If you have difficulty locating this muscle or using the techniques above, look for a weighted vaginal cone, which may be available in stores/websites where intimate products are sold.

Health Risks Associated with Menopause

The onset of menopause increases the risk of other health conditions for women, namely osteoporosis, heart disease, and Alzheimer's disease. It is important to be aware of these health risks, since preventive strategies can be implemented.

Osteoporosis

Explained in greater length in Chapter 13, osteoporosis is a condition in which bone mass deteriorates, resulting in thin, weak, and brittle bones. Not all women develop osteoporosis, despite the accelerated bone loss associated with menopause. A woman who enters menopause with a high bone density will be less likely to develop osteoporosis because she starts off with more bone. Still, menopause has been identified as a risk factor for osteoporosis; estrogen plays an important role in maintaining healthy bones, and its declining levels can contribute to bone loss.

Heart Disease

Estrogen production during the reproductive years provides protection against heart disease. This hormone increases good cholesterol (HDL) levels and reduces triglyceride levels. It also has positive effects on the blood vessels, as both a vasodilator (opens up the blood vessels) and an antioxidant. Some of this protection is lost during menopause because of estrogen deficiency.

Alzheimer's Disease

Symptoms of Alzheimer's disease include loss of memory, impaired judgement and reasoning, and changes in mood and behavior. While the exact causes of Alzheimer's are unknown, estrogen deficiency as it occurs in menopause has been linked to memory loss and the deterioration of cognitive function. Some studies have found that women taking estrogen replacement therapy have a lower risk of Alzheimer's disease,[2] but the research is conflicting.

Managing Menopause

There is no "one size fits all" treatment for menopause. Every woman is unique, with her own symptoms, family history, health risks, views, and goals. The management of menopause must therefore be tailored to the individual woman.

Hormone Replacement Therapy

Hormone replacement therapy (HRT) refers to the use of estrogen and progesterone to supplement or replace hormones whose levels decrease in menopause. Women who have undergone a hysterectomy are given estrogen on its own. Other women receive progesterone in conjunction with estrogen, to protect the uterus. HRT is available in pills, creams, gels, and patches, and a variety of regimens can be followed.

In the past, doctors recommended HRT for most women. Today's practitioners are more reluctant to prescribe hormones because of known side effects and health risks. Such a decision involves many factors: among them, the age of the woman, the extent of her menopausal symptoms, her risk factors for heart disease, osteoporosis, and breast cancer, and her personal feelings about HRT.

Benefits of HRT

- *Relief of symptoms.* HRT use often results in rapid and effective alleviation of hot flashes, mood swings, skin and vaginal dryness, and other menopausal symptoms.
- *Prevention of osteoporosis.* A well-documented benefit of estrogen is its ability to prevent, arrest, and potentially restore bone loss. Since most bone loss occurs within five to seven years after menopause, HRT treatment should be started early if it is to be used for this reason.

- *Reduced risk of colorectal cancer.* Estrogen offers protection against colorectal cancer. A recent study indicated that it reduces the risk of death by this cancer by 20 to 50 percent.[3]
- *Alzheimer's disease.* Estrogen has a protective effect on the brain and enhances memory and cognitive function. Some studies have suggested that estrogen replacement may help prevent and treat Alzheimer's disease owing to its antioxidant properties and its ability to enhance cerebral blood flow.

Risks of HRT

- *Side effects.* Approximately 5–10 percent of women experience undesirable side effects, including nausea, breast tenderness, headaches, and bloating. Many of these side effects are dose related.
- *Increased risk of breast cancer.* One of the most recent studies to look at this issue, the Women's Health Initiative (WHI), found that women were at an increased risk of developing invasive breast cancer after 3 years of HRT use. This risk increased with the duration of use and was greatest for those taking HRT for 10 years or longer.[4]
- *Endometrial (uterine) cancer.* Estrogen taken on its own by women who have a uterus can increase the risk of endometrial cancer five- to tenfold.[5] Progesterone taken in conjunction with estrogen counters this effect and reduces the risk of endometrial cancer.
- *Heart disease.* It was previously thought that HRT offered heart protection, but recent studies indicate HRT may actually increase the risk of heart attack, stroke, and blood clots.[6]
- *Gallbladder disease.* Estrogen pills taken by mouth can increase the risk of gallbladder disease requiring surgery by 48 percent.[7]
- *Liver disease.* HRT should be avoided by those with liver disease because a healthy liver is needed to metabolize hormones properly.

Bio-identical HRT

There has been great interest in the past few years in "natural" rather than synthetic hormones. Natural hormones are identical to those produced by the body, hence the term bio-identical. These products are not commercially available and therefore must be made by a "compounding pharmacist" (compounding pharmacists have specialized training in the preparation of pharmaceuticals—they make creams, lotions, capsules, etc.). Clinical research on these products is limited, but many practitioners believe they are safer than synthetic hormones and, in theory, provide the same benefits as the body's own hormones.

Natural Products for Menopause

While HRT offers certain benefits, it is not right for everyone. But whether a woman chooses to take HRT or not, she can still adopt any of a number of complementary approaches that may ease the symptoms of menopause and improve overall health. Some of these approaches may also reduce the risk of diseases such as cancer, heart disease, and osteoporosis.

Vitamins and Minerals

Even women who eat a balanced diet can benefit from vitamin and mineral supplements. Alcohol use, smoking, stress, HRT, anti-epileptic drugs, and emotional disorders all increase a woman's need for vitamins. Vitamin and mineral supplements can serve as an "insurance policy" against possible deficiencies, optimizing health. The following are some of the particularly helpful vitamins and minerals for menopausal women:

- *Multivitamin/mineral complex.* This should be the foundation of a woman's nutritional program, ensuring that basic needs are met. Look for a product that has 50–100 milligrams of the B vitamins, with antioxidants (beta carotene, C, E, selenium, zinc) and minerals. The B vitamins help to manage stress, anxiety, and depression.
- *Calcium/Magnesium/Vitamin D.* These help to maintain bone density, build strong bones, and reduce the risk of fracture. Supplements of calcium and vitamin D can enhance the bone-sparing effects of estrogen.[8] Calcium and magnesium also reduce stress and promote relaxation.
- *Vitamin E.* As an antioxidant, vitamin E may offer protection against heart disease by preventing oxidation of plaque in the blood vessel walls and preventing blood clotting. It may also alleviate hot flashes and skin and vaginal dryness. Furthermore, a recent study showed that women who took vitamin E over a two-year period reduced their risk of fatal heart attacks by 40 percent.[9] The recommended dosage is 400–1,000 IU daily.
- *Antioxidants.* These nutrients combat free-radical damage and may reduce the risk of heart disease and cancer. Look for the network antioxidants: vitamins C and E, glutathione, lipoic acid, and coenzyme Q10. Antioxidants work better when taken together because they recycle and enhance each other's action.

Herbal Approaches

For decades, herbal medicines have been used to manage menopause around the world. In North America, these therapies are gaining in popularity and acceptance within the medical community. Many herbs are promoted in the treatment of menopausal symptoms, but research is strongest for black cohosh and soy. Other products (red clover, chaste tree berry, ginkgo biloba, St. John's wort, and wild yam) may offer benefits for specific symptoms, but research is limited.

Black cohosh   Black cohosh is popular worldwide for managing menopausal symptoms, but it is not fully understood. In some clinical studies, it has been compared to prescription estrogen and found to be just as effective in the management of hot flashes, night sweats, insomnia, nervousness, and irritability.[10] Though rare, side effects include abdominal pain, nausea, headaches, and dizziness. Black cohosh is sometimes used to help women wean off estrogen supplements; this should be done under a doctor's supervision. The dosage is 20–40 milligrams daily. Look for a product standardized to contain 2.5 percent triterpene glycosides.

Chaste tree berry   Chaste tree berry is commonly used in the management of PMS, but it also alleviates perimenopausal symptoms. This herb balances fluctuating hormone levels and regulates the menstrual cycle.[11] Women with irregular or heavy menstrual bleeding or cyclic breast swelling may benefit. The recommended dosage is 175 milligrams daily. Look for a product standardized to contain 0.5 percent agnuside and 0.6 percent aucubin, the main active ingredients. Chaste tree berry can interact with medications that modulate dopamine levels in the brain (e.g., certain antidepressant and antipsychotic drugs) and should be used cautiously by people taking these drugs.

Cranberry   Cranberry has a long history of use for maintaining healthy urinary tract functions. It was originally thought that cranberry worked to kill bacteria by acidifying the urine. It has now been proven that the cranberry contains unique compounds called proanthocyanidins, or condensed tannins, that prevent bacteria from adhering to the bladder wall, allowing the body to flush these infectious organisms away.

Drinking cranberry juice is not the most efficient way to reap the benefits of cranberry. The amount required is quite large (32–64 ounces), since stomach acids destroy the tannins. That would add a lot of calories to your diet and be costly. Scientists have developed a concentrated extract of cranberry, called Cran-Max®, which is clinically proven to be a safe and effective treatment for reducing the occurrence and severity of infections. This formula utilizes a delivery system called Bio-shield®, which protects the cranberry fibers from being destroyed by the stomach and helps increase cranberry's absorption. One capsule of a product providing 500 milligrams of Cran-Max® daily is an effective dose. This product is very safe and well tolerated.

Ginkgo biloba   Ginkgo biloba helps improve memory and cognitive function and has been proven effective for blood vessel insufficiency and age-related decrease in brain function. Ginkgo increases blood flow and oxygen delivery to the brain. It is also a potent antioxidant, preventing free-radical damage in the brain, eyes, and heart. Look for a product containing the extract EGB 761, such as Ginkoba®. Start with 40 milligrams three times daily with meals. Be cautious if you're taking blood thinners or Aspirin, since ginkgo can enhance the effects of these drugs. Consult with your doctor because of the possible increased risk of bleeding when multiple anticoagulants are taken.

Ginkgo biloba has been approved in Germany for the treatment of Alzheimer's disease. In one study, specific extract of ginkgo biloba (EGB 761) was found to stabilize and, in many cases, improve mental and social functioning with use of six months to one year.[12]

Red clover extract   Red clover contains a high concentration of isoflavones. It's been suggested that it improves menopausal symptoms, but more research is needed in this area. Research on its cardiovascular benefits has been conflicting. One trial found that red clover improved systemic arterial compliance (a measure of the elasticity of the arteries) but had no effect on cholesterol levels.[13] The usual dosage of red clover is a standardized extract providing 40 milligrams of isoflavones daily. Red clover has blood-thinning properties, so should be used cautiously by those taking blood thinners. If you use blood thinners, consult with your doctor before taking red clover.

St. John's wort   St. John's wort is commonly used for depression. Several clinical studies have found it as effective as prescription drugs in the treatment of mild to moderate depression, without the side effects.[14] The recommended dosage is 300 milligrams three times daily. Look for a product standardized to contain 0.3 percent hypericin, the active ingredient. St. John's wort is a very safe product with few side effects, but it can interact with other antidepressants, immunosuppressants, and oral contraceptives, so consult with your doctor if you are taking these medications.

Valerian root   Because of its mild sedative properties, valerian root improves the quality of sleep and the amount of time spent in deep sleep.[15] It's quite safe and doesn't cause dependence, addiction, or next-day drowsiness. Some people experience a headache with its use. The recommended dosage is 300–500 milligrams one hour before bed. Don't combine valerian with prescription tranquilizers or sedatives.

Wild yam   Wild yam is commonly used to treat menstrual disorders and menopausal symptoms. Products containing wild yam are often promoted as providing a source of progesterone, but this is a false claim. Wild yam cannot be converted into progesterone by the body, but it may offer other health benefits. Preliminary research suggests that it increases HDL cholesterol[16] and supports the adrenal glands. The latter effect would be important in the early stages of menopause, since the adrenal glands kick into action to produce hormones after the ovaries shut down their production.

Combination Formulas

Rather than taking a variety of supplements for menopause, some women prefer a combination formula that addresses various health issues. These formulas can help manage menopausal symptoms, regulate hormone levels, and reduce risk factors for chronic diseases such as heart disease and osteoporosis. Read the labels carefully to ensure that you are getting therapeutic doses, and look for products that have been clinically tested. Two such products that we recommend are Natural HRT™ by Swiss Herbal Remedies and Estrologic™ by Quest Vitamins.

Functional Foods

As we learned in Chapter 7, functional food contains value beyond basic nutrition. Foods such as soy, flaxseed, garlic, and broccoli reduce menopausal symptoms and cardiovascular risk factors.

The isoflavones in soybeans mitigate hot flashes, slow down bone loss, lower cholesterol, and possibly protect against breast cancer.[17] Most experts recommend about 60 milligrams of soy isoflavones daily, in divided doses. This would amount to approximately 7 ounces of uncooked tofu, 2 cups of cooked or canned soybeans, or 1/3 cup of roasted soy nuts.

Flaxseed is a rich source of fiber, omega-3 fatty acids, and lignans. Preliminary research suggests that flaxseed may offer protection against breast cancer.[18] Fiber keeps the bowels regular, reduces the risk of colon and breast cancer, and lowers cholesterol. HRT users should add extra fiber to their diets because it helps the body eliminate hormones more efficiently. Omega-3 fatty acids reduce risk factors for heart disease by reducing cholesterol levels and lowering blood pressure. Lignans, a type of plant-derived estrogen found in food such as flaxseed, soy, and legumes, may help alleviate menopausal symptoms. To receive all the health benefits of flaxseed, take 1–2 tablespoons of milled flaxseed daily.

Lifestyle Interventions

Women should keep in mind that lifestyle choices have an effect on their health during menopause.

- Soy and flaxseed aren't the only foods that offer benefits to the menopausal woman. Raw fruits and vegetables, garlic, onions, nuts, seeds, and whole grains are others. Boost your broccoli intake, especially if you are taking HRT, since it is a good source of fiber, antioxidants, and minerals and also contains a chemical that helps break down estrogen. Broccoli may also offer protection against breast cancer and heart disease.

- Eating about 30 grams of fiber daily helps regulate mood, curb appetite, and reduce the risk of heart disease and certain cancers. Avoid processed food and fast food.
- Stress can make menopausal symptoms more pronounced. Meditation, yoga, and focused breathing have been shown to decrease the frequency and severity of hot flashes and to strengthen one's sense of well-being.
- Regular, moderate physical activity improves a woman's physical and emotional well-being during menopause. Exercise stimulates the release of endorphins (happy hormones), relieving stress, anxiety, and depression. Clinical studies have proven that exercise reduces the frequency and severity of hot flashes.[19] It is also important for a healthy heart and healthy bones.

Here are some other strategies you'd do well to keep in mind:

- Dress in layers. Peel clothes off during a hot flash. At night, remove extra blankets or sheets when you feel hot.
- Avoid spicy food. Food like hot peppers can worsen hot flashes.
- Do not smoke. Smoking can contribute to anxiety, irritability, and depression.

Conclusion

Menopause and perimenopause represent a transition in a woman's life. While the symptoms can be uncomfortable, they are manageable. One of the most difficult decisions a woman must make during this time is whether or not to take HRT. This is an individual decision for each woman, one that must take into consideration her own symptoms, health risks, and personal desires. Mounting research supports the use of herbs, nutritional supplements, and lifestyle changes as means to relieve menopausal symptoms, reduce the risk of chronic disease, and improve quality of life. Women need to take a proactive approach to the management of their health in menopause by researching their options and asking questions. From greater knowledge and awareness comes a feeling of control; thus empowered, women will find it possible to enjoy health and vitality during menopause.

16

MEN'S HEALTH: FUNCTIONING SOUTH OF THE BORDER

Most men ignore the early warning signs of poor health, but two health issues seem to grab their attention: the enlarged prostate and waning sexual function. Men do well to pay attention, since prostate anomalies and poor sexual performance frequently accompany other health problems. This is because many of the factors that cause enlarged prostate and sexual decline are also responsible for other age-related diseases.

Below we will discuss the typical changes seen in the aging man. We will look at the impact of diet, lifestyle, and stress on a man's health. And we will outline what can be done to prevent and treat the most common conditions.

The Prostate

A man's prostate gland is located underneath the bladder and behind the urethra, which carries urine out of the body. It reaches its mature weight of 20 grams when a man is 20. The function of this walnut-sized gland is to add secretions to the ejaculatory fluid that improve the quality and motility of sperm and thus increase a man's fertility. The prostate is also responsible for lubricating the urethra and thereby protecting it from the irritating contents of urine.

Prostatitis

Since the prostate connects to the urethra, bacteria and other microbes can travel from the urinary tract and infect this delicate gland. *Prostatitis* is an inflammation of the prostate gland, likely caused by microbial infection. For instance, men can contract infections of the prostate through unprotected sex. Drinking too much alcohol and caffeine (local irritants for the urinary tract) and consuming refined sugars (which weaken immune function) also contribute to increased susceptibility to infection in the prostate. Remarkably, chronic or invasive infection originating in the gut, the lungs, or the lymphatic system can also produce prostatitis.

Untreated, chronic infection of the prostate can lead to serious problems. These include reduced fertility, urinary tract infection, and kidney damage. If prostatitis is suspected, the man and his sexual partner need to be assessed by a doctor. The following list contains some of the common signs and symptoms of prostatitis. If any of them apply to you, see your doctor.

- Decreased volume of urine due to blockage of urinary tract
- Low back pain
- Burning pain or discomfort when voiding urine
- Blood or sediment in urine
- Low-grade fever, chills, or fatigue
- Increased daytime or nighttime urinary frequency
- Hesitating when urinating
- Pus-like or milky secretions from penis
- Excessive dribbling
- Inability to empty bladder completely
- Pain in groin or scrotum
- Impotence
- Strong odor and/or dark, concentrated urine
- Despite urgency, unable to void urine

Benign Prostatic Hyperplasia (BPH)

The majority of men will some day have to deal with *benign prostatic hyperplasia* or *hypertrophy*. In BPH, the prostate gland becomes progressively enlarged, reaching three to five times its normal weight (in extreme cases as much as ten times). The incidence of BPH is 10 percent of the male population in their thirties, 70 percent of men in their sixties, and an incredible 90 percent of men in their seventies. Almost every man over 80 (90–95 percent of them) has some degree of BPH. Clearly, BPH is an age-related phenomenon.[1]

As the prostate gland grows larger, the flow of urine is obstructed and urine is retained in the bladder longer than is normal; this increases the likelihood of infection anywhere in the urinary tract—kidneys, bladder, and urethra. The most serious complication of untreated BPH is kidney damage. Over time the bladder becomes over-stretched and loss of muscular control ensues, making it difficult to empty the bladder completely. The signs and symptoms of BPH overlap considerably with those of prostatitis.

Nevertheless, it's important to be familiar with signs that may indicate BPH. These symptoms, too, should be reported to your doctor.

- Increased urinary frequency, particularly at night
- Dribbling
- Decreased force and/or calibre of urinary flow
- Pain when voiding urine
- Difficulty starting or, once it begins, stopping urination
- Floating tissue or scrapings of the urethra in the urine
- Urine that is cloudy, dark, or has a strong and unusual odor

All men in their forties or at least by the age of 50 should have their prostate examined for significant enlargement. If you are uncomfortable with the procedure, discuss with your doctor the usefulness of ultrasound as a diagnostic tool. Don't let fear or embarrassment hold you back—an undetected problem can lead to severe complications. Also, since prostate cancer is the most common cancer among men, speak to your doctor about getting a prostate-specific antigen (PSA) test done. This simple blood test detects whether any cancerous process has begun in the prostate. Slight to moderate elevations of PSA often indicate BPH, while significant elevations, particularly in younger men, indicate prostate cancer in about 90 percent of the cases. Cancer is always more successfully treated when detected early.

Testosterone

To get a basic understanding of the causes of BPH, we need to look at the masculine (or "bravado") hormone testosterone. Below is a list of the main functions of testosterone when optimal levels are maintained.

- It maintains muscle mass and bone density.
- It is responsible for sexual desire and function.
- It elevates and stabilizes mood.
- It optimizes brain function (concentration and memory).
- It aids in the burning of fat.
- It maintains cardiovascular health.
- It regulates cholesterol and triglycerides.
- It regulates blood pressure, blood-sugar, and insulin levels.
- It is responsible for fertility.
- It maintains connective tissue and skin elasticity.
- It maintains energy levels and improves endurance.

When men reach about 35, their blood levels of unbound or free-form testosterone (the most beneficial form) decline and they can expect to see many changes in their health. The most common changes are a loss of lean body mass and bone density and a decline in energy, physical strength, stamina, and sexual function. As they age, many men find that fat accumulates in their abdominal region (forming the "potbelly") and that they suffer from loss of memory, lack of concentration, moodiness, and irritability. Because of declining testosterone levels, the aging man is also at increased risk of age-related diseases like heart disease, stroke, diabetes, hypertension, obesity, arthritis, and osteoporosis.

Unfortunately, replacing what was lost with testosterone supplements is no solution, since testosterone accumulates in the prostate during the aging process—in most cases to the detriment of the gland. The testosterone that is concentrated in the prostate is converted to dihydrotestosterone (DHT), and DHT is 10 times more potent than testosterone when it comes to stimulating tissue growth in the prostate. To make matters worse, the enzyme responsible for the conversion of testosterone into DHT (5-alpha-reductase enzyme) becomes more active during the aging process. Thus, increased production of DHT is a major factor in BPH.[2] Incidentally, high levels of DHT are also responsible for hair loss.

Stress and BPH

Stress is the major factor responsible for both declining testosterone levels and age-onset BPH. As we've discussed, stress causes cortisol to rise sharply during the aging process, and consistently elevated levels of cortisol cause the hypothalamus-pituitary-adrenal (HPA) stress axis to remain engaged and to be incapable of shutting down. This isn't a good situation, since too much testosterone is produced with the HPA axis constantly turned on. And what happens to you when you have excessive cortisol, adrenaline, and testosterone in your system? You can feel overly aggressive, hostile, easily annoyed, and extremely frustrated by the smallest of things. (Yes, men—not just women—are sometimes at the mercy of out-of-control hormone fluctuations.) However, while stress initially encourages the overproduction of testosterone (contributing to enlargement of the prostate), eventually the body simply gets exhausted and can no longer meet the excessive demand for testosterone; at that point, testosterone levels decline.

Insulin resistance is another common consequence of stress-induced high cortisol levels, and it too leads to BPH. (Excessive stress, lack of exercise, and overindulging in carbohydrates, sweets, and alcohol all contribute to the development of insulin resistance.) Your potbelly and the loss of muscle mass on your arms can all be blamed on insulin resistance. Moreover, as fat accumulates in the abdominal region, more aromatase (a bad enzyme) is produced. Aromatase converts testosterone to estrogen; hence, high levels of aromatase lead to a decline in testosterone and a rise in estrogen. Elevated estrogen has been implicated in the development of BPH.[3]

Overweight aging men typically have elevated estrogen levels. Rising estrogen levels cause an increase in the production of a protein known as *sex hormone-binding globulin* (SHBG). SHBG is no friend to the aging man, since it binds to the beneficial free-form testosterone, making it less available to the rest of the body. The aging man, then, especially one who's overweight, ends up with higher estrogen and lower testosterone levels. Therefore, higher levels of SHBG have also been implicated in BPH.

Environmental Exposure and BPH

Many scientists firmly believe that the worsening chemical soup of our environment is a major factor in hormonal imbalances in both men and women.[4] For instance, xenoestrogens are environmental chemicals (for example, plastic resins and pesticides) that mimic estrogen stimulation in the body. Excessive estrogens—whatever their source—spell trouble. In men, excessive estrogen reduces fertility, impairs sexual function, worsens BPH, and increases the likelihood of prostate cancer.

Your liver carries the burden of detoxification, so be good to it. The liver removes toxic testosterone by-products such as DHT, excessive estrogens, SHBG, and xenoestrogens. Coupled with declining testosterone levels, all these hormonal aberrations greatly contribute to BPH and poor sexual function in the aging man. Thus, if you keep your liver healthy, you'll be taking a huge step towards keeping your hormones in balance, having good overall health, and avoiding serious complications of BPH.

Drinking too much alcohol on a regular basis eventually impairs the liver's ability to balance hormones. It also depletes nutrient levels, increases abdominal weight, and is directly correlated with BPH complications. Apparently, the worst type of alcohol is beer. The hops in beer have a hormone-stimulating effect on the prostate gland, leading eventually to enlargement.[5]

Too many of us continue to pollute our environment and ourselves with cigarettes. Cadmium is one of the many dangerous chemicals in cigarettes, and smoking leads to higher levels of cadmium in the body. Cadmium is a toxic heavy metal that interferes with zinc absorption and function. This has a terrible effect on the male body, since zinc not only helps maintain a healthy immune system, but also balances male hormones and ensures prostate health.[6]

Diet and BPH

A man's diet can have a huge impact on his health. A research study showed that a high-protein diet containing 44 percent protein, 35 percent carbohydrates, and 21 percent fat inhibits the activity of the enzyme responsible for enlargement of the prostate (5-alpha-reductase enzyme, which converts testosterone to DHT). The same study indicated that the opposite is also true: a low-protein diet (10 percent protein, 70 percent carbohydrates, and 20 percent fat) was shown to stimulate the activity of the 5-alpha-reductase enzyme.[7]

In general, increasing protein while reducing carbohydrates and fats is a good way to regulate insulin and blood-sugar levels, since high levels of the two latter are common in diseased aging. As we've seen, high insulin levels are linked to an enlarged prostate. Furthermore, high insulin levels impair proper detoxification of toxic testosterone metabolites, estrogens, and SHBG. Successfully managing stress and gaining dietary control of blood sugar will positively influence testosterone levels and metabolism.[8]

Although it's a good thing to increase dietary protein, it is not advisable to consume a 44 percent protein diet on a regular basis. If necessary, this level may be maintained for a few weeks to a couple of months at a time to regulate blood sugar and control weight. However, a safer maintenance amount would be anywhere between 25 and 35 percent. Furthermore, it's important to eat a variety of both animal and vegetable protein. This means eating lean beef, chicken, turkey, fish, eggs and beans, nuts, seeds, and soy foods.

You should also consume high-fiber foods—whole grains, vegetables, and fruits. Fiber helps to rid the body of bile that is laden with toxic hormone metabolites, and it's thus a great help to the liver. In disposing of bile, fiber also helps to remove excessive amounts of cholesterol. When cholesterol is high and antioxidants (vitamin C, E, beta carotene, selenium) low, free radicals can do more damage to cholesterol, causing it to become oxidized (much like butter turning rancid after being left on the counter overnight). Oxidized cholesterol blocks arteries and causes circulatory problems in the heart and the rest of the body. Moreover, high amounts of oxidized cholesterol are extremely toxic and carcinogenic with respect to the prostate because they contribute to excessive cellular growth. Thus, lowering cholesterol levels while increasing antioxidant levels helps control age-related BPH and its complications.

Like all age-related diseases, BPH is a chronic inflammatory disorder. A diet that's rich in essential fatty acids (omega-3 and omega-6) helps the body control inflammation. A diet high in saturated fats—steak, eggs, bacon, cheese, and milk—fuels the inflammatory process. Thus, diets high in protein obtained solely from land animals increase the progression of BPH and affect overall health. Refer to the discussion on inflammation in Chapter 10.

Ways to Maintain or Achieve Prostate Health

Let's now look at some things you can do to have a healthy prostate, maintain sexual function, and ensure overall health as you age.

1. Find ways to cultivate a positive mental attitude, and learn to cope better with stress. Plan for sufficient rest and relaxation each and every day. Think of ways to have fun. Go to bed at a reasonable time and get seven to eight hours of quality sleep. Engage in exercise (strength training, aerobics, and stretching) for 30 minutes three to five times a week. If you smoke, quit—there's lots of help if you need support. Drink no more than 2 cups of coffee a day or 3–5 alcoholic drinks a week. Get to or maintain an ideal body weight. Go over the various chapters in this book that cover these topics.

2. Take a look at your diet. Make sure you're getting 30–40 grams of fiber daily from fruits, vegetables, whole grains, nuts, seeds, and beans. If this is difficult, consider using supplemental powdered fiber daily. Fresh-ground flaxseeds, one of the best sources of fiber, promote hormonal balance in many ways. Drink 6–8 glasses of pure water daily. Your body needs adequate water and fiber to detoxify and cleanse itself. Pumpkin seeds

contain essential fatty acids, protein, vitamins, and very high levels of zinc and other minerals; these nutrients nourish the prostate gland. Eat high-quality, nutrient-dense foods at least three times daily at regular times. Review the information on diet, digestion, and cleansing in Chapter 9.

3. Take a high-quality multiple vitamin and mineral supplement three times each day. Make sure you're getting 30–45 milligrams of elemental zinc daily; it has favorable effects on male hormonal balance, prostate health, and sexual function; insufficient amounts are directly associated with low blood levels of testosterone, low quantity and quality of sperm, and low volumes of semen. Take 800 IU of vitamin E and at least 1,000 milligrams of vitamin C daily to get antioxidant support. Make sure you get at least 50 milligrams of vitamin B6 daily (100–200 milligrams daily if you have severe BPH-related complications). Among many important functions, vitamin B6 improves protein metabolism, elimination of water and waste, and hormonal balance. Because of its antioxidant and anti-cancer properties, 200 micrograms of selenium should be taken daily. An optimal amount of 800 IU of vitamin D should also be taken daily; this vitamin improves calcium metabolism and participates in hormone regulation and cancer prevention. Two tablespoons daily of Udo's Oil is one of the better ways to get a balanced intake of essential fatty acids in order to control inflammation of the prostate and all tissues of the body. Essential fatty acids also improve cardiovascular health, and good circulation is needed for optimal sexual function. Review the material on diet, inflammation, and essential fatty acids in Chapter 10.

4. Visit your doctor regularly for a complete physical examination and the appropriate laboratory tests. Talk to your doctor about evaluating the health of your prostate. If BPH has been diagnosed and treatment is necessary, consider the options outlined below.

Plant-Based Medicines for Benign Prostatic Hyperplasia (BPH)

Saw Palmetto

A daily dose of extract of saw palmetto berries (320 milligrams standardized to contain 85–95 percent fatty acids) has been shown to prevent enlargement of the prostate and to decrease the size of the gland in moderate cases. At least 20 clinical trials have shown that saw palmetto is effective in BPH, improving poor urinary flow and reducing frequency.[9]

Stinging Nettle

Stinging nettle leaf and root are rich in a variety of vitamins, minerals, fatty acids, and antioxidant compounds. Stinging nettle can be regarded as a tonic for the urinary tract because of its diuretic and anti-inflammatory properties. It is also useful for the prevention and treatment of gravel in the kidneys, thus helping prevent kidney stones. In addition to improving urinary flow, it addresses the factors that lead to prostate enlargement. Evidence suggests that it may help to increase free-form testosterone levels. It is best to consult with a professional for optimal daily dosages of stinging nettle.[10]

Pygeum Africanum

Pygeum africanum extract is derived from the bark of an evergreen tree native to South Africa. An extract of the plant improves prostate gland secretions, thereby boosting the fertility rate and providing better lubrication for the urethra. *Pygeum* also improves urinary flow, reduces frequency, and provides relief for pain or irritation during voiding of urine in cases of BPH. Moreover, it has been shown to increase a man's capacity to have an erection where this ability is hindered by BPH or prostatitis. The effective dosage of standardized *pygeum* would be 100–200 milligrams daily.[11]

Pollen Extract

A special extract of flower pollen, derived primarily from rye and sold under the trade name Cernilton or Prostaphil-2™ (available from Advanced Orthomolecular Research; see Appendix 7.1), has proven effective in the management of BPH. Some studies have shown that this extract improves all measurements of good urinary flow; others, that it reduces the size (both weight and volume) of the prostate. Moreover, clinical studies have shown benefits with prostatitis.[12]

Soy

Both soy protein and soy extracts are of great benefit in the prevention and treatment of BPH as well as in the overall health of men. Soy protein helps to control cholesterol levels and reduces the risk of cardiovascular disease. The consumption of 20–80 milligrams of isoflavones (soy-derived compounds commonly referred to as phytoestrogens) is believed to be the main reason why the incidence of BPH-related problems and prostate cancer is significantly less in the male population of Japan than in that of North America. Research suggests that men should consume 20–30 grams of soy protein containing at least 20 milligrams of phytoestrogens daily.[13]

Green Tea and Lycopene

Green tea and green tea extracts with high amounts of polyphenols (beneficial compounds) improve the body's ability to detoxify, neutralize free radicals, and prevent the oxidation of cholesterol. Ongoing research is also validating green tea's anti-cancer properties.

Lycopene extract (the pigment in tomatoes that makes them red) is an extraordinary antioxidant and anti-cancer compound. Higher levels of lycopene in men's tissue are linked to (among many things) a lower incidence of prostate cancer.

Research data about green tea and lycopene strongly suggest that both should be included in the diet and in a comprehensive supplemental program to ensure good health and provide protection for the prostate.

Indole-3-Carbinol (I3C)

Broccoli, Brussels sprouts, and cabbage are rich sources of indole-3-carbinol (I3C). Available as a dietary supplement, this powerful phytochemical helps maintain estrogen balance. It also helps detoxify excessive and toxic forms of estrogen and promotes their excretion out of the body (it's thus a great help to the liver), thus preventing them from causing excessive tissue growth. Given its numerous roles, I3C can be regarded as an anti-cancer compound. For men with significant BPH or at risk of prostate cancer, daily doses of 400–500 milligrams of I3C should be considered.[14] (See Appendix 7.1.)

Treatment Options for BPH

When prescription medication is carefully selected and monitored, it can be effective in the treatment of BPH. The medication can be expensive, however, and the side effects that may accompany it—impotence and loss of libido—are unacceptable to many. Throughout Europe, phytomedicines (plant-based medicines) are used as first-line therapies for BPH, far outstripping their prescription counterparts in usage and effectiveness. Should you decide to use phytomedicines to prevent or treat BPH, ask an experienced professional to help you select the one that's best for you. However you choose to address your prostate concerns, you must not attempt to bypass the lifestyle and dietary recommendations made above. Equally important, your doctor should monitor your progress to help you evaluate the success of any chosen therapies.

Treatment Options for Prostatitis

Once prostatitis has been diagnosed, antibiotics are routinely prescribed for weeks at a time, giving only temporary or little relief. This is often because there are other causes of prostatitis besides microbial infection. Significant stress is a major factor in chronic inflammation of the prostate as well as in the urinary constriction seen in prostatitis.

Cernilton or Prostaphil-2™, the flower pollen extract mentioned above, is a good choice for chronic prostatitis. A variety of phytomedicines (dandelion, golden rod, corn silk) improve urinary flow, control inflammation, and soothe an irritated urinary tract. Men who suffer from chronic recurring urinary tract infections that can lead to prostatitis may want to consider Cran-Max®, a standardized extract of cranberries that may help to reduce the incidence of infection. Check with a professional before selecting a plant-based medicine for your treatment.

Ways to Improve Sexual Performance

Most men are turning to prescription medication to improve sexual performance, since results are significant in most cases. This approach should always be coupled with improvements in lifestyle and diet, as sexual difficulties usually signal the existence of other problems. Impotence is sometimes the result of depression, but in most cases the culprit is stress-related fatigue, BPH, obesity, high blood pressure, poor circulatory health, or uncontrolled blood sugar. No aging man should expect to have a healthy sex life if he can't control or reduce his stress level, eat a proper diet, get enough sleep, and exercise regularly. And if sexual intimacy is to be gratifying, the aging man needs to have a harmonious and fulfilling relationship with his partner.

Many phytomedicines are effective in treating impotence and have other benefits as well. Cordyceps, for example, a mushroom extract, improves lung and kidney function and acts as a restorative tonic for the whole body. This natural product is highly revered in China for its usefulness in treating physical and mental exhaustion, especially the kind of exhaustion that accompanies long-term illness. Cordyceps can also improve cardiovascular function, immune function, sleep, and stamina. Reliable evidence also shows that it is a great benefit to men who suffer from impotence, premature ejaculation, physical weakness, and stress.[15] Organika's Cordyceps Mushroom is made to exacting standards and contains the therapeutic compounds that bring the multiple benefits mentioned above. (See Appendix 7.1.)

Conclusion

It should be clear to the aging man wishing to function south of the border that he needs to address all areas of his health. A good diet, regular exercise, a positive mental attitude, and emotional balance are all critical. A lot has been said in this and other chapters about how you can achieve this healthy lifestyle. While many nutritional supplements and phytomedicines have been recommended, taking them is of little use if that's all you do. You can only avoid age-related problems, including benign prostatic hyperplasia and sexual decline, if you adopt a well-rounded healthy lifestyle. The aging man who has already developed health problems can do many things to improve his situation. The acquisition of sound knowledge needs to be followed by action.

17

KEEPING YOUR MARBLES

Everyone faces an inescapable fact about aging: the brain is vulnerable to the passage of time. Still, you have a choice. You can either slow down the brain-aging process or you can let the process slow you down. Life's journey can be particularly unkind to the cells of the brain and the rest of the nervous system. The first thing you might notice is short-term memory failure. You might joke, "I must be losing my marbles." Humor is good medicine, but you need much more than that to forestall age-related changes in the brain.

Advanced cognitive decline, senile dementia, Alzheimer's, Parkinson's, and stroke become increasingly common as people age. Most older people quietly suffer a chronic, low-grade depression that goes unrecognized. Many experience insomnia. Loss of physical coordination and vertigo put aged individuals at great risk of injury through falling. Individually or collectively, these problems can be debilitating.

The good news is that current research shows that most of the negative changes seen in the aging brain can be successfully prevented and perhaps even treated. To help you understand how to stay mentally agile, we will first describe the general structure of the brain. Then we will identify some of the negative factors that affect brain function. Finally, we will outline therapies that protect and enhance brain function, and discuss treatments for depression and neurological diseases.

General Structure and Function of the Brain

Over 100 billion nerve cells (neurons) form over a million trillion connections in the brain, and these cells need to be fed. The brain consumes roughly 20 percent of the oxygen taken into the body and 25 percent of the body's glucose to sustain function. On average, by age 50, most people experience a 20 percent drop in blood flow to the brain. This drop continues as people age, which means that less and less oxygen, glucose, and other nutrients is delivered to the starving brain cells. Insufficient blood flow is due to poor circulatory health, and poor circulatory health, in turn, is largely due to cardiovascular disease, diabetes, obesity, smoking, and physical inactivity.

The brain is responsible for all intelligent thought (it reasons, makes rational decisions, learns, stores and retrieves information, and so on). The right and left sides of the brain are symmetrical in size, but in most people one side or the other is dominant, producing distinct traits. Left-brained individuals tend to be skilled in science, mathematics, reading, and verbal communications. Their decisions are guided by logic or reasoning. Right-brained people are often insightful, perceptive, creative, artistic, musical, and socially oriented. Their decisions are guided by emotions and intuition. Although North American society generally measures intelligence by left-brain function, success in life has little to do with which side is dominant.

Measuring Intelligence

The brain allows us to experience the world physically through the five senses of smell, taste, touch, sight, and sound. We can process the world intellectually and emotionally as well. A person can be said to have integrated intelligence when the intellectual and emotional functions of the brain are balanced and well integrated. Our ability to make decisions and learn from experience depends on this balance. A well-integrated intelligence is believed to be the major factor enabling people to reach healthy ages of 100 or more.[1]

Negative Influences on the Aging Brain

Stress

Many factors inhibit the development or maintenance of the well-balanced brain. By now, no one should be surprised to learn that stress is the most significant of these. Specifically, excessive or prolonged exposure to stress raises cortisol levels. This stress hormone literally fries your brain, singeing billions of brain cells. The part of the brain most vulnerable to cortisol damage is the limbic system; this system contains several glands, including the hippocampus, hypothalamus, and pituitary. Commonly referred to as the emotional brain, the limbic system governs, among other things, mood, memory, and sleep.

Prolonged exposure to stress (i.e., to high cortisol levels) can cause insomnia, memory failure, depression, and burnout. A high cortisol level is in fact one of the hallmark features of depression-related problems. Furthermore, when the brain floats in a sea of cortisol, blood sugar becomes erratic, exacerbating depression. The brain needs a steady supply of glucose, and even the slightest fluctuation in blood sugar can throw off brain function. Everyone—not just diabetics—needs to have tight control of blood sugar to maintain optimal brain function.

On a cellular level, when there's an excess of cortisol, too much calcium gets into the brain cells. As calcium accumulates in the aging brain, there is a progressive drop in energy, decreased neurotransmitter production, increased inflammation and free-radical production, and an accumulation of toxins in the brain cells. When brain-cell damage is pervasive, serious neurological diseases develop, such as Parkinson's and Alzheimer's. Autopsies of people with Alzheimer's disease typically show significant brain calcification. Calcification plus insufficient blood flow spells an increased risk of stroke.

Stiffening of the Brain

A diet too rich in sugar can make brain tissues stiffer and thereby slow down metabolism. A stiff brain makes it harder to think clearly, and it predisposes you to all sorts of neurological diseases. Trans fatty acids also stiffen the brain. Formed when oils are fried or hydrogenated, trans fatty acids occur in high amounts in french fries, margarine, snack foods, and other processed foods—that is, in foods that are also high in refined carbohydrates and sugar.

Death by Overstimulation

Excitotoxicity, a process whereby brain cells are stimulated to death, is the term used to describe how excessive cortisol destroys brain cells. An excitotoxin is any substance, whether produced by the body or derived from environmental sources, that is capable of stimulating brain-cell function. Two food additives that have been implicated as excitotoxins are monosodium glutamate (MSG) and aspartame. Continuous exposure to these and other excitotoxins ultimately stimulates brain cells to death.[2]

Alcohol and Caffeine

A lifetime of excessive alcohol and caffeine consumption also accelerates brain aging. While it's true that drinking a moderate amount of wine may be beneficial, your brain doesn't need alcohol to operate. Most healthy individuals over the age of 100 do not consume alcohol.[3]

While caffeine may keep you alert and enable you to think more quickly, it doesn't improve mental performance. In fact, too much caffeine will increase the number of mistakes made and ultimately slow down work productivity. Caffeine magnifies feelings of stress by raising levels of cortisol and adrenaline. It makes things seem much bigger than they really are. Over the long haul, caffeine can cause memory impairment, depression, anxiety, insomnia, and nerve damage in the brain. If you need caffeine, drink no more than 2 cups, or 16 ounces, daily and forgo the sugar.[4]

Food Sensitivities

Most people aren't aware that sensitivities to certain foods can alter brain function. Sensitivities to dairy products and refined grains—especially wheat—manifest as mental confusion, depression, anxiety, hyperactivity, and obsessive-compulsive disorders.[5] Basically, these and other food proteins sedate or excite the brain by preventing neurotransmitters from working properly.

Problems in the Liver and Gut

Also underestimated is the effect of the liver and gut on brain function (see discussion in Chapter 9). The gut digests and absorbs the food that will eventually feed your brain. Enough enzymes need to be produced and released into the gut to break protein down into amino acids. The brain uses these acids to make the neurotransmitters that ensure proper functioning of the body. All this activity is threatened during the aging process, since digestive enzymes become depleted.

In leaky gut syndrome, the liver exhausts itself trying to process toxins that leak through the intestinal walls. These poisons eventually accumulate in the blood and break down the blood–brain barrier. When this barrier is weakened, poisons are easily deposited in the brain, causing headache, forgetfulness, and scattered thinking.

Depression

Many of the above factors can manifest as depression. If you are constantly worried and can't relax or experience joy, you may have one of the many forms of depression. Take a look at the signs and symptoms of depression listed below. See your doctor if you experience most of these. Medication is sometimes initially required to lift more serious forms of depression.

- A change in appetite that causes weight gain or weight loss
- Insomnia or hypersomnia (desire to sleep a lot)
- Physical inactivity or hyperactivity
- Feeling anxious, nervous, scared, worried, and easily overwhelmed most of the time
- Feeling angry or annoyed with oneself or others most the time
- Feeling burdened with things most of the time; unable to relax
- Feeling hopeless or worthless; negative self-image; excessive or inappropriate guilt or shame

- Loss of interest in life; decreased sexual desire
- Inability to think or concentrate
- Loss of energy and feelings of fatigue
- Recurrent thoughts of death, suicide, or attempted suicide

Therapies for the Brain

The Plastic Brain

No matter what state your brain is in now, it can be changed. There was a time when the brain was viewed as a static lump of mush, that all brain damage was irreversible. Not true. One of the most exciting aspects of the brain is its ability to grow new cells and increase the number of connections. This has been well documented in stroke and other cases of brain damage. The brain's ability to restore function by bypassing (rewiring around) sites of injury is known as its neuroplasticity.[6]

We now think of the brain as being neuroplastic; that is, with proper physical and mental stimulation and nourishment, it can be remolded or reshaped. The brain grows through proper use and support at any age. Unfortunately, chronic stress is the wrong kind of stimulation. Lower your stress and you'll lower your cortisol, and in the process you'll give your brain the best rejuvenating tonic it could ask for. Let's now take a look at some specific things you can do to help your brain.

Achieving Optimal Brain Function

1. Learn to recognize what stresses you. Simplify stress by identifying what you can and cannot control.

2. Make an appointment with yourself each day to get in touch with your true feelings; share them with friends and family.

3. Be aware of how you speak to yourself in stressful situations. Stop trying to be perfect. Acknowledge your mistakes and take corrective action. Then forgive yourself.

4. Learn to relax. Deep breathing and meditation are excellent ways to ease tension. Take the time to sit quietly and practice these techniques every day.

5. Don't let fear hold you back. Pursue your interests. Find things to get excited about. Develop a sense of purpose and passion. Only through trial and error can you discover who you are and what you really want.

6. Learn to laugh and don't take yourself too seriously. There is so much humor in life. Finding it is only a matter of changing your perspective.

7.   Learn to love and accept yourself first and foremost. Express your love to the people in your life and show them your appreciation.

8.   Get to bed and wake up at a regular time. The brain needs a good night's rest, about seven to nine hours—much more than previously thought. There are many safe and non-addicting supplements that promote sleep. Also, take periodic rests daily to give your brain a break.

9.   Engage in different forms of exercise (stretching, walking, biking, swimming, weightlifting) three to five times a week to improve circulation. Engage in mental exercises, too (reading, crossword puzzles, board games, brain teasers, math problems without a calculator).

10. Eat a wholesome diet and eliminate food to which you are sensitive. Higher intake of nutrient-dense foods and higher blood levels of antioxidants and B vitamins in the elderly translate into better cognitive performance and memory.[7] Also drink at least 6 glasses of pure water daily to make sure your brain is well hydrated.

Developing a Supplement Program

To develop a supplement program that will help your brain, you need to identify your own particular needs. To manage stress and regulate blood sugar, see Chapter 8. To optimize digestion and cleanse the body, see Chapter 9. To control the damaging effects of age-related inflammation in the brain, see Chapter 10. We present more general recommendations below. But again, anyone on prescription medication should consult a qualified health-care provider before beginning a vitamin and mineral program.

- Take a well-balanced, high-quality vitamin and mineral supplement three times daily with each meal.
- Make sure you get about 800 milligrams of calcium, 400 milligrams of magnesium, 20 milligrams of zinc, 200 micrograms of selenium, 200 micrograms of chromium, and all the B vitamins daily.
- Have your doctor measure your homocysteine level and make sure it is between 4 and 8. (Homocysteine is a waste by-product of protein metabolism that can cause poor circulation and brain toxicity; it has been linked to many neurological diseases.) If your homocysteine level is high, increase your intake of folic acid, B6, and B12.
- Take 400–800 IUs of the kind of vitamin E that includes all the tocopherols.
- Take 1,000–2,000 milligrams of vitamin C.
- Take 2 tablespoons of Udo's Oil daily. This is one of the best ways to get a balanced intake of the essential fatty acids that control inflammation and improve cell-membrane fluidity and brain function.

- Take 60–180 milligrams of coenzyme Q10, which offers protection against free-radical damage and improves energy production in brain cells.

Other Therapeutic Supplement Considerations

Methylcobalamin

If you are over 50, have your doctor assess your vitamin B12 levels. Since this vitamin is not easily absorbed from dietary and supplement sources, your doctor might want to give them to you by injection. An alternative to injections is a sublingual (dissolved under the tongue) preparation of vitamin B12 known as *methylcobalamin*. Methylcobalamin is poorly stored in the body, and when it is at low levels, neurological symptoms such as numbness, tingling of hands and feet, and depression are seen, even if blood levels of the regular form of B12 are adequate. This is because during aging not enough regular vitamin B12 is converted into methylcobalamin. Methylcobalamin protects the brain against stress and a variety of toxins, and can actually help heal damaged neurons. It helps those with diabetic neuropathy, Alzheimer's, Parkinson's, multiple sclerosis (MS), and other serious neurological diseases. Five milligrams sublingually of methylcobalamin twice daily should be enough to enhance brain function. Doses of up to 60 milligrams daily may be required in advanced cases of neurological disease.[8] (See Appendix 7.1.)

Ginkgo Biloba

Ginkgo biloba extract helps prevent free-radical damage and improves blood flow, thus aiding oxygen and glucose distribution to any part of the body, including the brain. One emerging benefit of ginkgo is that it appears to protect the delicate areas of the brain that are responsible for mood, memory, and mental performance against age-related or stress-induced damage. In one particular study involving patients with a variety of dementias (including Alzheimer's), Ginkoba (a standardized extract of ginkgo biloba; see Appendix 7.1) was shown to halt progression of the disease and improve cognitive performance and social function in a significant number of cases.[9] It may also be helpful in preventing or treating age-related tinnitus, vertigo, macular degeneration, memory failure, and depression. Typical doses of standardized gingko are 120–240 milligrams daily.

Citicoline

Citicoline, or CDP-choline, a naturally occurring compound produced in the body, is available as a supplement. Citicoline protects the brain from over- or under-excitation and acts as a traffic cop in ushering nutrients into and pumping waste out of the brain cell. This compound enhances the synthesis of acetylcholine and dopamine, two very important neurotransmitters involved in mood, memory, and mental performance. It also helps with the production of energy and protects the brain from damage caused by poor circulation and low oxygen levels. It may be helpful for the recovery of stroke, depression, age-related cognitive decline, dementia (including Alzheimer's), Parkinson's, and other neurological diseases. Citicoline taken orally is well absorbed and crosses the blood–brain barrier. Typical doses are 500–1,000 milligrams daily.[10] (See Appendix 7.1.)

Phosphatidylcholine (PC) and Phosphatidylserine (PS)

Other options to citicoline are phosphatidylcholine (PC) and phosphatidylserine (PS). They are similar in that they help improve brain-cell integrity and metabolism. Both are prepared from soy lecithin. PC helps with acetylcholine production and with fat and cholesterol metabolism, and protects the liver and gut from toxic damage. It benefits those with liver and gastrointestinal diseases, elevated cholesterol levels, Alzheimer's disease, and bipolar depression. Typical doses of PC are 2–12 grams daily. Make sure that at least 35 percent of the soy lecithin preparation is phosphatidylcholine.[11]

PS is most concentrated in the cells of the brain, and thus it is thought to play a critical role in optimal brain function. Perhaps because of the aging process or because of nutrient insufficiencies, the PS production declines as we age. Low levels of PS are typically seen in elderly people suffering from depression and poor mental function. PS supplements have helped aged individuals with problems related to memory, concentration, learning, and mood; PS has also helped them adapt better to stress. PS is believed to make brain cells more responsive, increase the number of brain-cell connections, and protect the brain from the damaging effects of stress-induced cortisol. Thus, PS benefits people with poor mental function, depression, and dementia-related neurological diseases. Typical doses of PS are 100 milligrams three times daily.[12] (See Appendix 7.1.)

S-Adenosyl-L-Methionine

S-adenosyl-L-methionine (SAM) is a universal amino acid used by the body to improve the quantity and quality of brain cells; it is involved in the production of all the major neurotransmitters. SAM also helps with the production of connective tissue, possesses anti-inflammatory properties, and aids the liver in detoxification. It is helpful in lifting depression and alleviating arthritis and liver disorders. Typical daily doses of SAM are 400–1,600 milligrams.[13] Be sure to take a high-quality multiple vitamin and mineral supplement that includes all the B vitamins, since these vitamins improve the activity of SAM.

St. John's Wort

In recent years St. John's wort extract has become by far the most popular naturally derived product used for mild to moderate depression. This phytomedicine alleviates the symptoms of depression just as well as the common prescription medications, but without the side effects. It also helps those with stress-related anxiety, muscle tension, and insomnia. St. John's wort should not be mixed with prescription antidepressants without medical supervision. Typical doses are 300 milligrams, standardized to contain 0.3 percent hypercin, three times daily.[14]

Valerian

Valerian is believed to calm jittery nerves, relax muscles, and help those with mild to moderate insomnia. It should be used with caution during the day because, depending on the dose, it may act as a sedative. Ideally, a health-care practitioner should investigate the causes of ongoing anxiety and insomnia before valerian is used on a long-term basis. It should never be mixed with other prescription or over-the-counter medications used for sleep. Typical doses are 200–1,000 milligrams of standardized valerian, either spread throughout the day or taken at bedtime.[15]

Conclusion

A lifetime of chronic or poorly handled stress, poor nutrition, and an unhealthy lifestyle spells brain deterioration and leaves you with very little to enjoy in your advanced years. If you nurture your brain, however, you can be mentally active and happy in every stage of life. Recognize your brain's many needs. The scores of natural products for cognitive function and emotional balance are of little value if you rely on them alone. You must integrate what has been outlined in this chapter to ensure good brain health during the aging process. Foremost, seek to achieve mental and emotional harmony within yourself and with those around you. When you have a loving relationship with yourself and others, the brain's chemistry will give you an incredible and enduring passion for life.

PART 4

THE THREE BIGGEST HEALTH CONCERNS RELATED TO AGING

18

HEART DISEASE: FOLLOWING A NEW BEAT

Cardiovascular disease (CVD) is our biggest killer! We all recognize the importance of a healthy heart to our health and longevity, but statistics indicate that this knowledge has not persuaded all of us to take better care of our hearts. Roughly 40 percent of all deaths in North America are attributed to CVD,[1] making it the number one killer on this continent. An estimated 61.8 million Americans have some form of CVD, and more than 725,000 of them die as a result each year.[2] In Canada, it is estimated that roughly 8 million people have CVD, from which (extrapolating from 1999 data) about 79,000 will die.[3] As might be expected, the incidence of CVD mortality rises with age, but a significant number of those deaths still occur in the under-65 age group. For people looking for longer active lives, we are not doing a very good job of pursuing our dream. Let's take a look at the known risk factors and learn what we can do to protect our hearts.

Risk Factors

An estimated 63 percent of Canadians have at least one of the three major modifiable risk factors associated with CVD—smoking, high blood pressure, and high blood cholesterol.[4]

- *Smoking.* Smoking reduces oxygen supply, starving the working heart muscle of its all-important fuel and making it work harder to move blood through the body. The nicotine in tobacco makes the heart beat faster, narrows blood vessels, and thus increases blood pressure. In the long term, nicotine leads to an accumulation of plaque in the blood vessels, permanently increasing blood pressure and the chances of clotting and an eventual stroke.[5]

- *High blood pressure.* Also known as *hypertension*, high blood pressure has been linked to family history, ethnicity, chronic stress, excessive alcohol consumption, obesity, and, of course, smoking. Blood pressure is also age related; the incidence of high blood pressure is more than 50 percent higher in the 65–74 age group than in the 35–64 age group.[6] Our chance of developing high blood pressure increases if either of our parents experienced it or if there is a greater incidence of the condition in our ethnic background. More in our control, however, are the hypertension risk factors of chronic stress, excessive alcohol consumption, and obesity.

- *High blood cholesterol.* Forty-three percent of Canadians are living with elevated cholesterol levels. Family history, liver dysfunction, lack of exercise, and eating too many saturated fats all contribute to this problem. The result is an increased risk of heart disease.[7]

Older people are more apt to have at least one of the major modifiable risk factors listed above, but when other major risk factors are included—sedentary lifestyle, obesity, and diabetes—nearly half of Canadians between 18 and 34 years old have at least one major risk factor and the figure jumps to more than 70 percent for those in the 35–64 age bracket.[8] The sedentary nature of many of today's jobs and the addictive nature of television and the Internet contribute to the collective lethargy so common in North American society. Being overweight puts additional strain on the heart, and the link between hypertension and obesity has been widely noted—more than 75 percent of people with high blood pressure are overweight.[9] Though diabetes is not as common a risk factor as those mentioned, it, too, is a serious contributor to heart disease nonetheless.

One risk factor that has only recently been identified is high blood levels of *homocysteine*, a naturally occurring amino acid found in the body. Those with the highest levels of homocysteine in their blood have a greater risk of death from coronary artery disease.[10] Another recently discovered risk factor is the presence of *lipoprotein (a)*, also known as Lp_a, the stickiest form of "bad" cholesterol, which greatly increases the buildup of cholesterol in blood vessels.[11]

Diagnosis

A number of tests can help determine whether or not you have CVD. Non-invasive tests include chest X-rays, electrocardiograms, echocardiograms, exercise stress tests, computed tomography scans, and magnetic resonance imaging (MRI) or angiography (MRA) tests.[12] More invasive tests include thallium stress tests, multiple-gated acquisition (MUGA) scans, single photon emission computerized tomography (SPECT) tests, and positron emission tomography (PET) scans.[13]

Screening

Major risk factors for heart disease can be identified by blood tests for HDL (good) and LDL (bad) cholesterol levels, as well as for triglycerides. Recently, a blood test was developed to determine levels of C-reactive protein in post-menopausal women, another symptom of higher risk of heart attacks and strokes. Nearly all of us have had our blood pressure checked at one time or another, and this is a straightforward way to determine whether or not we have that telltale risk factor.

If you are concerned that you might be a candidate for CVD, early detection is a key factor in decreasing the odds of your suffering a debilitating or even fatal heart attack or stroke. Talk about your concerns with your doctor.

Treatment Options

Many drugs can be used to deal with the risk factors in heart disease; some reduce blood pressure and cholesterol, others prevent clotting and strengthen the pumping of the heart. For some of us, these drugs are essential for quality of life and even for life itself, but they aren't the sole answer to this vast problem. We hope this book has been showing you that you must move beyond just drugs and surgery to fix your problems. You can only break the age barrier with an integrative approach, one that combines conventional and complementary therapies with heart-healthy lifestyle choices. Regular exercise and a heart-healthy diet, along with other complementary therapies (vitamins, minerals, and herbs), not only help prevent but also help treat heart disease.

Exercise

Regular aerobic exercise decreases your chances of developing heart disease by strengthening your heart and limiting the major contributing risk factors. However, less than half of us make exercise a regular part of our lives.[14] The National Institutes of Health suggest that you accumulate at least 30 minutes of moderate physical activity almost every day in order to protect yourself from heart disease.[15]

The results of regular exercise can be impressive. One study indicated that women who regularly walked at a moderate pace for at least one hour per week were half as likely to develop CVD as those who did not exercise at all; the longer the duration of walking each week, the more promising were the results.[16] Another study indicated that those who expend the most energy per week in physical activity and vigorous physical activity are the least likely to develop coronary heart disease.[17] People who are already living with heart disease or who are recovering from a heart attack or stroke can also benefit from exercise, reducing the likelihood of their death during rehabilitation by as much as 25 percent.[18]

Cardiac Cuisine

Chapter 7 detailed the fundamentals of nutrition for optimal health. Some foods, however, are more specifically beneficial for the heart than others. The aim of a heart-healthy diet is to cut back on saturated fats and cholesterol and increase consumption of essential fiber, fruits, and vegetables. Of course, we should cut back on alcohol, salt, and the sweet-but-empty calories of candy, soft drinks, and other junk food. Daily consumption of some functional foods, like soy products, garlic, and flaxseed, can significantly decrease our cholesterol and triglyceride levels.

Eating more fish is also beneficial. Mounting clinical research has shown that the omega-3 fatty acids found in fish oil (EPA and DHA) can lower blood pressure and reduce atherosclerosis.[19] Most studies found benefits with 3 grams of omega-3 oil per day (that is, 10 grams of fish oil). The best results were found with 15 grams per day, nearly impossible through diet. Supplements were thus often recommended. Some evidence suggests that high doses of fish oil (3 grams daily) after a heart attack can reduce the risk of a second episode.[20]

It's best to pass on coffee and instead try green tea; it contains antioxidants (polyphenols) shown to lower total cholesterol levels and improve the ratio of LDL to HDL.[21] Most of the research is based on the amount found in the typical Asian diet (3 cups per day).

Supplements for Heart Disease

Numerous nutritional supplements help in the treatment and prevention of heart disease. Keep in mind that these supplements are not intended to replace prescription medication. In most cases, they can be taken along with prescribed therapies, but it's always wise to check with your doctor or pharmacist to avoid any negative interactions.

Vitamin E

Vitamin E is an antioxidant that works to prevent oxidation of LDL cholesterol and also helps to prevent blood clotting. Some studies have found that people who take at least 100 IU of vitamin E per day have a lower risk of heart disease.[22] However, a few recent studies have cast some doubt on the benefits of vitamin E. One of them—the HOPE trial, which looked at the effect of vitamin E in preventing heart attack in older patients at a very high risk of heart attack[23]—did not show any benefit in supplementing with 400 IU of vitamin E. It is unclear why this and other studies contradict the findings of the majority. One possibility is that vitamin E works to prevent LDL cholesterol oxidation, an effect not measured in these contradictory studies.

Most practitioners still feel that vitamin E is beneficial for heart health, and it is certainly very safe. The usual recommended dose is 400–800 IU daily. Be aware that vitamin E enhances the blood-thinning effect of certain drugs (Aspirin and warfarin).

Vitamin C

As an antioxidant, vitamin C works to protect LDL cholesterol from oxidative damage.[24] The body also uses it to produce collagen, a substance that strengthens blood vessels.[25] People with higher blood levels of vitamin C seem to have lower blood pressure.[26] This effect may be due to the ability of vitamin C to enhance the activity of nitric oxide, a chemical needed to dilate blood vessels and prevent spasms. The usual recommended dose is 500–1,000 milligrams daily, but some studies suggest heart protection can be attained with doses as low as 100 milligrams per day.[27] Smokers need extra vitamin C, as smoking depletes vitamin C levels in the body.

Antioxidant Complexes

Studies have also looked at the benefits of antioxidant complexes. Blood levels of the antioxidant vitamins A, C, E, and beta carotene tend to be lower in people with a history of heart attacks.[28] In these people, the number of damaging free-radical molecules is higher, suggesting a greater need for antioxidants. In a large study involving heart attack victims, it was found that vitamins A, C, E, and beta carotene significantly reduced infarct size (the area damaged by heart attack).[29] Many manufacturers offer antioxidant complexes, and formulations vary. Read the labels carefully to ensure that you are getting a therapeutic dose. One product that we recommend is Protect+ by Greens+. This formula contains vitamins C and E and beta carotene, along with other nutrients that aid heart health, including selenium, coenzyme Q10, and grape seed extract.

B Vitamins

Several of the B vitamins offer heart protection. Niacin (vitamin B3) lowers cholesterol levels,[30] though higher doses can cause flushing and stomach ache. Another form of niacin, inositol hexaniacinate, is much more easily tolerated and offers benefits similar to those of cholesterol-lowering drugs.[31] The usual starting dose is 500–1,000 milligrams three times daily.

B vitamins offer other benefits as well. Preliminary studies have shown that vitamin B6 can reduce the risk of blood clotting and lower blood pressure. Vitamins B6 and B12 and folic acid lower homocysteine levels.[32] While the exact amount of these vitamins required to lower homocysteine levels is not known, most practitioners recommend 25–75 milligrams of vitamin B6, 100–1,000 micrograms of B12, and 400–1,000 micrograms of folic acid. People with digestive disorders or malabsorption syndromes (celiac disease) or who use certain drugs (antacids, anticonvulsants) are at a higher risk of B-vitamin deficiency.

Calcium

Many of us think of calcium as a nutrient for bone health, but this mineral is also important for the proper functioning of our muscles, especially the heart muscle. A calcium intake (through diet or supplements) of 800–1,500 milligrams per day has been found to lower blood pressure.[33]

Calcium supplements may also help to lower cholesterol. Preliminary research has found that 1–2 grams per day provides some benefits.[34] Different forms of calcium vary greatly in their absorption and tolerability. Calcium citrate is a preferred form, since it is easily absorbed, better tolerated than the carbonates, and more affordable. Calcium supplements should be taken with meals, and the daily dose split up if it is greater than 500 milligrams.

Magnesium

Magnesium is involved in energy production (i.e., in the manufacture of ATP [adenosine triphosphate], the energy source for the body), muscle relaxation, and many other critical body processes. Magnesium status can affect the heart in different ways. It has been found that people who die of heart attacks have lower magnesium levels. Traditionally, injectable magnesium has been used as a treatment for acute heart attack. It reduces the risk of heart damage and death by dilating the coronary arteries, thereby improving oxygen delivery to the heart, reducing the heart's workload, preventing blood-clot formation, and improving heart rhythm.

A deficiency of magnesium has been linked to low HDL cholesterol levels (undesirable), while supplements have been shown to lower total cholesterol.[35] High levels of magnesium (350–600 milligrams per day) can lower blood pressure.[36]

Magnesium deficiency is common, especially among those who have a poor diet, drink too much alcohol, or use diuretics, oral contraceptives, or estrogen. Supplements are particularly beneficial in lowering blood pressure in people taking diuretics, as these drugs reduce magnesium (and potassium) levels in the body.[37] Supplements also benefit people with heart conditions such as angina, mitral valve prolapse, cardiomyopathy, and congested heart failure. The usual range for supplementation is 600–1,200 milligrams daily.

Selenium

Selenium is a trace mineral that offers many health benefits as an antioxidant. It protects us from the toxic effects of heavy metals such as lead, mercury, and aluminum, and the body uses it to produce glutathione peroxidase, an even more potent antioxidant.

Some research suggests that a selenium deficiency increases the risk of heart attack and that supplements are helpful in reducing that risk.[38] Smokers with low selenium levels may be at particular risk.[39] In a study in which selenium was given along with coenzyme Q10 to people who had suffered a heart attack,[40] it was found that the antioxidants reduced the risk of a second heart attack.

While severe selenium deficiency is rare, marginal deficiencies are commonly reported in North America. Depleted soil conditions are partly to blame, since the selenium content of grains and vegetables is dependent on that in the soil in which they are grown. Certain drugs (histamine [H2] blockers and proton pump inhibitors, which are used to reduce stomach acid) reduce selenium absorption. The usual supplement dosage is 100–400 micrograms daily. Doses greater than 1,000 micrograms can cause problems—loss of fingernails, skin rashes, and changes in the nervous system.

Coenzyme Q10 (CoQ10)

CoQ10, also known as ubiquinone, is found throughout the human body. It is an essential component of the mitochondria (energy powerhouse) of all of our cells and is thus involved in the process of converting food into ATP. It also works as a powerful antioxidant and helps to preserve vitamin E.

CoQ10 is particularly concentrated in the heart and offers numerous benefits for heart health. Studies have shown that it can significantly lower blood pressure,[41] as well as levels of Lp_a cholesterol.[42] One study involving heart attack survivors showed that 120 milligrams per day reduced the risk of a second episode and death in a subsequent episode.[43] CoQ10 has also been shown to help people with congestive heart failure, cardiomyopathy, and angina.[44] CoQ10 levels tend to be lower in older and/or overweight individuals and in those with hypertension, cardiomyopathy, and heart failure. It has been suggested that these conditions increase the body's use of CoQ10, explaining the depletion. The cholesterol-lowering drugs lovastatin, pravastatin, and simvastatin also deplete CoQ10 levels. The usual dose of CoQ10 for heart health is 50–200 milligrams daily, taken with meals. This is a very safe supplement with no known side effects.

Policosanol

Policosanol is a mixture of waxy substances manufactured from sugarcane. Numerous studies have shown that policosanol can substantially improve cholesterol levels, with effects comparable to the most effective drugs.[45] It appears that policosanol works in the liver to slow down cholesterol synthesis and increase liver reabsorption of LDL cholesterol.[46] It also seems to have blood-thinning properties similar to those of Aspirin.[47] In studies involving more than 1,000 patients, policosanol was effective in reducing LDL cholesterol by at least 20 percent and total cholesterol by about 15 percent.[48] Some studies found that it raises HDL cholesterol and lowers triglycerides.

The recommended dose to lower elevated cholesterol is 5–10 milligrams twice daily. The best results were obtained at higher doses of 20 milligrams daily. It may take two months or longer to see the benefits. Look for a product derived from sugarcane, as there is no research supporting policosanol products derived from beeswax.

Policosanol appears to be safe at the maximum recommended dose. Mild, short-term side effects may include nervousness, headache, diarrhea, and insomnia. It should be used cautiously with blood-thinning drugs like warfarin and Aspirin.

Garlic

Garlic has long been used in the treatment of a variety of health problems, from colds to heart disease. There has been much debate over what its active ingredient is and which form—oil, powdered, or aged—is best. The majority of studies used aged garlic extract, Kyolic™. Researchers believe that the unique sulfur compounds in this product are responsible for its health benefits.

With respect to heart health, garlic can cause modest reduction of blood pressure, cholesterol, and triglycerides, and helps prevent blood clotting. It has been found that 600–900 milligrams of garlic extract daily, taken for at least four weeks, moderately improves blood pressure.[49] Other studies suggest that garlic can lower cholesterol by 9–12 percent over several months.[50] One study compared garlic with the cholesterol-lowering drug bezafibrate and found it to be comparable in efficacy.[51]

Garlic has been shown to help prevent atherosclerosis (the process whereby the arteries become clogged with plaque).[52] In a recently published four-year study, the effects of 900 milligrams of a standardized extract were evaluated in a group of people age 50–80. The garlic supplement was found to reduce arterial-plaque formation by 5–18 percent.[53]

Most practitioners recommend one to two cloves of raw, fresh garlic daily. For those who don't want the odour of garlic on their breath, aged garlic extract is recommended. The usual dose is 400–800 milligrams daily.

Guggul

Guggul is a traditional Indian medicine used for a variety of conditions, including high cholesterol. It is obtained from the sticky gum resin from the mukul myrrh tree. Several studies have demonstrated that guggul can lower cholesterol levels, and in India, it is part of the mainstream approach to atherosclerosis prevention. One study reported that guggul lowered blood cholesterol by 17.5 percent.[54] Another compared its effects with those of the drug clofibrate: the average fall in cholesterol levels was slightly greater in the guggul group; moreover, HDL rose in 60 percent of people taking guggul, while it didn't rise in those taking clofibrate.[55]

Most extracts contain 5–10 percent guggulsterones—the main active ingredient. The usual recommended dose is 100 milligrams of guggulsterones, taken in three or four divided doses. It may take 12 weeks or longer to obtain the benefits of guggul.

Oat Beta-Glucan

Numerous studies have demonstrated that oats can lower several risk factors for heart disease, namely high cholesterol and blood pressure, diabetes, and obesity. Oats contain one of the richest dietary sources of the soluble fiber oat beta-glucan. Numerous trials have found that three 28-gram (about 1 ounce) servings of oatmeal per day, providing a daily total of 3 grams of oat beta-glucan, reduces total cholesterol by an average of 6 milligrams per deciliter.[56] This is quite significant, given that a 1 percent reduction in blood cholesterol can reduce the risk of heart disease by 2–4 percent.[57] The evidence is so strong that the Food and Drug Administration allows the use of a "Heart Health" claim on products providing a minimum of 750 milligrams of oat beta-glucan in a serving.

There are several mechanisms by which oats lower cholesterol. Oat fiber forms a gel that binds bile acids and increases their elimination from the body. It is also felt that oats inhibit the formation of cholesterol and reduce its intestinal absorption. Oat beta-glucan can also be found in supplements. When choosing a supplement, look for products that contain Oat Vantage™. This standardized product contains 50 percent pure oat beta-glucan.

An Aspirin a Day ...

For years doctors have recommended Aspirin for prevention of heart attack and stroke in those who have had one of these episodes. Recent research suggests it may also help to reduce the risk of heart attack and stroke in those with no prior episodes. Aspirin prevents the early formation of blood clots, and people at high risk should not be surprised if their doctor recommends an Aspirin a day. There are side effects, however (stomach pain, nausea, dizziness, ringing in the ears, heartburn, and gastric bleeding), and since these are often dose-related, most doctors recommend the lowest effective dose, 81 milligrams daily.

Conclusion

Any effort you make to improve your health and increase your active longevity should start with the heart. Healthy eating, exercise, and stress reduction are all effective ways to avoid the major risk factors for heart disease. Maintaining heart-healthy practices may require some shifts in lifestyle, but this can be a positive experience and the results cannot be beaten—greater energy and a longer, more active life.

19

DIABETES: STOP
THE EPIDEMIC

Diabetes is a controllable and often preventable disease, yet it has become an epidemic in North America. In Canada, roughly 2 million people are affected;[1] in the United States, 17 million—and unfortunately, an estimated third of them don't know it.[2] While diabetes is not specifically age related, your risk of developing it increases as you get older. Roughly half of the reported diabetics are over 55 years old, and more than 20 percent of Americans over 65 are diabetic.[3]

The Escalating Incidence of Diabetes

The incidence of diabetes is growing at an alarming rate. From 1990 to 1998, the U.S. Center for Disease Control reported a 33 percent increase in the rate of diabetes among Americans, from 4.9 to 6.5 percent, and that rate rose another 6 percent in 1999.[4] The incidence in Canada has also escalated. Globally, the World Health Organization indicates that 150 million people are diabetic; this number is expected to be over 300 million by 2025, much of the growth occurring in developing countries. Most of the future diabetics in developing countries will be struck by the disease in the most productive years of their lives, between ages 45 and 64.[5]

Because diabetes is associated with other chronic diseases, these figures are especially troubling. It is estimated that 65 percent of diabetics die of heart disease or stroke, and do so at an earlier age than non-diabetics.[6] If left untreated, diabetes damages the kidneys, eyes, and circulation, and impairs immune function, reducing vitality and longevity.

Lifestyle and dietary practices significantly affect whether or not an individual will develop Type 2 diabetes. Non-diabetics and borderline diabetics can take steps to avoid the disease by watching their diet, monitoring their lifestyle, and, if necessary, supplementing with vitamins, minerals, and herbs. Diabetics can greatly reduce the disease's effects in much the same way.

Understanding Diabetes

Diabetes is a chronic disease in which the pancreas produces insufficient or ineffective amounts of insulin. Since insulin is critical in the processing of glucose into usable energy, a lack of it results in increased blood-glucose levels and a condition known as *hyperglycemia.*

There are two types of diabetes: Type 1 (formerly known as juvenile-onset diabetes or insulin-dependent diabetes) and Type 2 (formerly known as adult-onset diabetes or non-insulin-dependent diabetes).

Type 1 Diabetes

In Type 1 diabetes, the cells that produce insulin (called *beta cells*) become damaged or are destroyed. In infants and children, beta cells are usually destroyed rapidly, causing a sudden rise in blood-sugar levels. In adults, they are destroyed more slowly, causing a slower rise in blood-sugar levels.

The exact cause of Type 1 diabetes is unknown, but the standard explanation is that the immune system attacks and destroys the beta cells. People with Type 1 diabetes in their family history face a greater risk of contracting the disease. While lifestyle measures and supplements cannot correct the problem, they can help manage it by making the body more receptive to injected insulin.

Type 2 Diabetes

In the past, Type 2 diabetes was thought of as an adult-onset condition. The greatest increase of Type 2 diabetes in recent years however has occurred among children and adolescents.[7] Type 2 diabetes, the most common form of diabetes, occurs when the body stops producing enough insulin or, as is more often the case, the insulin produced is not properly utilized. The latter problem often starts when the body becomes resistant to the effects of insulin, a condition referred to as *insulin resistance.*

At the onset of Type 2 diabetes, the pancreas produces more insulin than usual after meals to try to compensate for the body's inefficiency, a condition known as *hyperinsulinemia.* Gradually, insulin secretion from the pancreas falters, and eventually stops, leading to full-blown diabetes. Risk factors associated with this type include a genetic predisposition, a poor diet, a sedentary lifestyle, being overweight or obese, ethnicity, and environmental factors.

The link between obesity and Type 2 diabetes is very strong. As many as 80 percent of people with Type 2 diabetes are overweight,[8] and to make matters worse, diabetes may itself increase the tendency to gain weight. Researchers now refer to these coexisting conditions as *diabesity*.

Early Warning Signs

The most common warning signs of diabetes include excessive thirst and hunger, frequent urination, fatigue, moodiness, frequent infections, and unusual weight loss.

Long-Term Health Risks

Over several years, the high blood-sugar levels associated with untreated diabetes can seriously damage nerves and blood vessels, resulting in vision problems, kidney damage, circulatory problems, and an increased risk of heart disease and stroke.

The likelihood of diabetics' developing these problems decreases if they manage the disease carefully. The Diabetes Control and Complications Trial, a decade-long study of more than 1,400 Type 1 diabetics in the United States and Canada, drove this point home in the early 1990s. The study participants, whose average age was 27 at the beginning of the project, were divided into two groups; one group underwent standard therapy treatments, while the other group undertook more intensive treatment to keep blood-glucose levels as close to normal as possible. Intensive treatment reduced the participants' risk of developing diabetes-related eye disease by 76 percent, kidney disease by 50 percent, and nerve disease by 60 percent. Researchers concluded that a reduction of blood-glucose levels like that experienced by the intensive-treatment patients slows the onset of these three diabetes-related complications and greatly reduces the risk of developing them at all.[9]

Prevention

Finding the dedication to follow recommendations for a healthy lifestyle isn't easy, but diet and exercise alone can make a significant difference. In one study, these two factors reduced the risk of developing diabetes by 31 percent among those who exhibited early signs of diabetes.[10]

Dietary Strategies

A balanced diet is crucial in the management and prevention of diabetes. There's no single perfect menu, but there are guidelines to follow and considerations to make when you decide what to eat. Some foods are definitely better than others for the maintenance of blood-sugar levels, and whenever you're in doubt, it's wise to seek advice from a registered dietician, one of the key people on the diabetes-prevention team.

The Carbohydrate Conundrum

Complex carbohydrates are a healthy choice for your diet—high-fiber whole grains (whole wheat, brown rice, oats, and flaxseed), along with legumes, beans, and vegetables. High-fiber foods are broken down more slowly and evenly, which helps to control blood-sugar levels. These foods also play a role in reducing cholesterol levels. Processed foods, containing refined sugars and flours, and foods high in starch are broken down more quickly, resulting in undesirable short, high bursts in blood-sugar levels.

The impact of foods on blood-sugar levels can be measured with the use of the *glycemic index* (GI). The GI provides a numeric measurement of the immediate effects of different foods on blood-glucose levels. Sugary and starchy foods are higher on the index scale because they cause sharp increases in blood sugar. High-fiber foods are lower on the scale because they have the opposite effect. Diets higher on the glycemic index are thought to increase the risk of developing Type 2 diabetes, while diets lower on the scale are associated with a lower risk.[11]

TABLE 19.1: Glycemic Index

LOW GLYCEMIC FOODS (GI < 55)

Almonds	Grapefruit	Peas
Apples	Kidney beans	Plums
Apricots	Lentils	Rice, wild
Barley	Milk	Soybeans
Bulgar	Oranges	Yogurt
Cherries	Pasta, whole wheat	
Chick peas	Pears	

MODERATE GLYCEMIC FOODS (GI 55–70)

Bran cereal	Honey	Rice, brown, basmati
Bread, whole wheat	Oatmeal	Sourdough bread
Buckwheat	Oatmeal cookies	Sweet potatoes
Carrots	Pita bread	Sucrose (table sugar)
Corn	Popcorn	
Grapes	Raisins	

HIGH GLYCEMIC FOODS (GI > 70)

Apricots	Dates, dried	Rice, short-grain, white
Baguette	Graham crackers	Rice cakes
Bananas	Kaiser rolls	Soda crackers
Bread, white	Mangoes	Soft drinks
Corn chips	Potatoes, baked	Watermelon
Corn flakes	Pretzels	

The GI of a food is influenced by several factors: the amount of carbohydrates it contains, the types of sugar found in it (glucose, lactose, sucrose), the type and quantity of starch, and the way it's cooked. Some ingredients (e.g., fats, tannins, and lectins) can decrease a food's GI because they slow the digestion process. However, the factor that most affects the GI is the amount of carbohydrates a food contains.[12] Recognizing this, most health authorities suggest that carbohydrates comprise 45–55 percent of total caloric intake. The Canadian Diabetes Association recommends that diabetics count carbohydrates and try to consume roughly the same amount of carbohydrates from meal to meal and day to day.[13]

Fiber

Oats have received a lot of attention in recent years. This common source of carbohydrates offers remarkable health benefits, reducing cholesterol levels, improving glucose levels, and reducing the risk of heart disease.[14] Most of the health benefits from oats come from beta-glucan, a soluble dietary fiber. When beta-glucan is consumed, it forms a gel that slows the digestion and absorption of nutrients, the result being a more gradual rate of glucose absorption.[15] The American Food and Drug Administration allows a "Heart Health" claim for oat products that provide a minimum of 750 milligrams of oat beta-glucan per serving. We can obtain up to 5 grams of beta-glucan fiber from 100 grams (about 3 ounces) of oatmeal and 7.2 grams from a similar serving of oat bran.[16]

For diabetics, oats can play a role in improving post-prandial (after meal) glucose levels and insulin response. Numerous clinical studies have demonstrated the benefits of oats on both fasting and post-prandial blood-glucose and insulin levels. Consuming between 6 and 8.4 grams of beta-glucan per day can reduce blood-sugar levels after meals by as much as 50 percent.[17]

Furthermore, according the Nurses' Health Study, a 10-year study of more than 75,000 American female nurses, regular fiber consumption is associated with a reduced risk of becoming diabetic and offers protection against heart disease.[18]

Sugar in Moderation

Years ago, the typical advice given to diabetics was to avoid sugar. Too much sugar or too many carbohydrates were thought to cause, or worsen, Type 2 diabetes. Eating a lot of sugary foods does increase blood-glucose and insulin levels, but most important is the total amount of carbohydrate calories (sugar or starch) we consume. Since sugary foods like candies and cookies lack nutritional value, we should eat less of them and choose healthier carbohydrate sources,[19] but we may not need to eliminate sugars entirely.

Protein

The recommendations for protein intake are the same for diabetics and non-diabetics: 20–30 percent of total calorie consumption, depending on activity level. Those with nephropathy (kidney disease) should limit their protein intake to 20 percent or less, depending on the severity of their condition.

Bad Fats

We all need to limit our consumption of saturated fats and dietary cholesterols. Since diabetics already have an increased risk of developing heart disease, it's important that they avoid dietary habits that exacerbate that risk. Diabetics are more sensitive to dietary cholesterol, so they should keep their saturated fat consumption below 10 percent of their total caloric intake and limit the amount of animal fat in their diets.

Friendly Fish Fats

Essential fatty acids (EFAs), like those found in some fish products, should be part of your regular diet. As explained in Chapter 7, foods containing EFAs are beneficial to heart health. By lowering triglyceride levels in Type 2 diabetics, EFAs (from food or supplements) provide some added protection for at-risk hearts.

The Value of Small, Frequent Meals

You can avoid accentuated highs and lows in blood-glucose levels by eating several small meals and snacks through the day rather than one or two large meals. By maintaining a steady blood-glucose level, you decrease the stress placed on your pancreas and thereby reduce your risk of developing, or exacerbating, Type 2 diabetes.

Weight Management

If you can maintain a healthy body weight, you have a better chance of avoiding diabetes (if you don't have it) or managing the disease (if you do). Excess body weight promotes insulin resistance, reducing sensitivity to insulin that the pancreas secretes and contributing to the onset of diabetes.[20] If you're overweight, shedding body weight and increasing your exercise regime can reduce insulin resistance and improve your maintenance of blood-sugar levels.[21]

Supplements

Nutritional supplements can help you control blood-glucose levels. Keep in mind, however, that you should use supplements under the guidance of a physician, pharmacist, or dietician.

Fiber Supplements

A simple way to gain greater control over blood-glucose and cholesterol levels is to increase fiber intake. Most health authorities recommend a minimum of 25 grams (about an ounce) of dietary fiber a day, a difficult amount to obtain through meals alone. There are a variety of fiber supplements; three quite beneficial types of supplements are psyllium, pectin, and oat bran.

Psyllium is found in many over-the-counter fiber supplements, most notably Metamucil™. It has been shown to reduce blood-glucose levels and total cholesterol.

Like psyllium, *pectin* slows the body's absorption of sugars and starches, helping to moderate blood-glucose levels. Found in many fruits, pectin can also be obtained as a nutritional supplement.

The benefits of *oats* can also be derived from supplements. Oat Vantage™, a commercially available supplement found in many products on the market, provides a concentrated amount of pure oat beta-glucan (50 percent).

Antioxidants

Vitamin E improves glucose tolerance in Type 2 diabetics[22] and helps reduce glycosylation.[23] Glycosylation refers to the damaging effect that sugars have on proteins in the body, affecting the function and health of all cells. As an antioxidant, vitamin E protects blood vessels from damage and may reduce diabetic complications like retinopathy (eye disease) and nephropathy (kidney disease).[24] It may take several months before the benefits of vitamin E supplementation are observable, and further studies are needed to determine whether vitamin E provides long-term protection against these complications. The usual recommended dosage is 400–800 IU daily.

Vitamin C improves glucose tolerance[25] and reduces glycosylation in Type 2 diabetics.[26] It has also been shown to lower blood levels of sorbitol, a sugar that can damage the eyes, nerves, and kidneys of diabetics.[27] Some doctors suggest that diabetics supplement with 1–3 grams of vitamin C per day (higher doses may cause diarrhea and increase blood-sugar levels).[28]

B Vitamins

Vitamin B6 (pyridoxine) and *B12* are important for the health of nerve cells. Vitamin B6 has been linked to improved glucose tolerance, as diabetics experiencing nerve damage have been shown to have low levels of B6 in their blood;[29] supplementation shouldn't exceed 500 milligrams per day unless under the advice of a physician, as higher doses can cause tingling in the extremities and other side effects. Vitamin B12 supplementation has been associated with reduced nerve damage and nerve pain in diabetics;[30] the usual recommended oral dose is 500 micrograms three times per day.

The body uses biotin, another B vitamin, to change glucose into glycogen (the stored form of carbohydrates). Like B6 and B12, biotin reduces pain from damaged nerves.[31] As well, biotin supplementation greatly reduces fasting glucose levels (i.e., levels after fasting, such as early in the morning before breakfast).[32] Doctors may prescribe 16 milligrams of biotin for a few weeks to see if blood-sugar levels will fall. While most multivitamins contain 50–100 micrograms of biotin per dose, the benefits mentioned here were achieved with much higher daily doses.

Chromium

Supplementation with chromium, a trace metal long touted as essential, improves glucose tolerance by increasing insulin sensitivity;[33] it may also lower total cholesterol, LDL cholesterol, and triglyceride levels,[34] reducing the risks of diabetic complications as a result. The usual supplemental dosages are 200–400 micrograms per day, though researchers use much higher doses in their studies.

Magnesium

Magnesium deficiency has been strongly implicated in insulin resistance and poor blood-glucose control, as diabetics tend to have low levels of magnesium in their blood.[35] Magnesium supplementation can help overcome this problem.[36] The usual recommended dosage is 300–400 milligrams per day. Since magnesium can cause diarrhea in higher doses, look for a supplement that combines it with calcium to offset that effect. Those with kidney disease should consult a physician before taking magnesium supplements.

Lipoic Acid

Lipoic acid is a naturally occurring antioxidant found in foods such as liver, yeast, and broccoli. It has been used for decades to regulate blood-sugar levels and prevent diabetic complications, such as neuropathy. Lipoic acid supplements improve glucose metabolism, insulin sensitivity,[37] and nerve health, and also reduce the negative symptoms of neuropathy in diabetics.[38]

Herbal Therapies

Bilberry, known for eye-health benefits, lowers the risk of cataracts and retinopathy in diabetics and may even treat the damaging effects of diabetic retinopathy.[39]

Ginkgo biloba, well known for its ability to improve circulation and blood flow to the brain, retina, and extremities, is used to prevent and treat nerve damage in diabetics.

Gymnema sylvestre, a plant native to southern India, has been used for centuries to lower blood-sugar levels in diabetics. It is thought that gymnema helps Type 2 diabetics produce insulin and that it improves insulin effectiveness in all diabetics. Current studies suggest that gymnema extract reduces the amount of insulin needed by Type 1 diabetics[40] and may eliminate Type 2 diabetics' need to take oral blood-sugar-lowering drugs.[41] With long-term use, gymnema curbs sweet cravings by numbing the taste receptors on the tongue. The typical daily dosage is 3–10 grams, in divided doses. Supplementation may require that you adjust your dosages of insulin or oral hypoglycemic drugs.

Asian, or *panax ginseng* has long been used to treat diabetes. Studies indicate that ginseng, like gymnema, aids the pancreas in the production of insulin, improves the body's use of that insulin,[42] and helps Type 2 diabetics control their blood-sugar levels.[43]

Conclusion

The incidence of diabetes is approaching epidemic proportions, and the traditional lines between juvenile-onset and adult-onset diabetes have become blurred in the process. It is important to recognize that the most prevalent form of the disease, Type 2, is strongly linked to lifestyle factors and that it can be largely prevented or, at the very least, controlled by a simple routine of exercise, healthy eating, and supplementation. There is thus little reason why diabetics cannot live longer and healthier lives than traditionally expected.

20

CANCER: GENETICALLY PROGRAMMED OR ENVIRONMENTALLY ACQUIRED?

Why is cancer more widespread today than at any other time in human history? Some think it is because people are living longer. True: cancer has become an age-related phenomenon. Others believe it has a lot to do with genetics. False: relatively few cancers (only about 5–10 percent[1]) are the consequence of "bad" genes.

Regardless of genetic makeup or family history, everyone risks sustaining the kind of damage to their genes that might result in the uncontrollable growth of cells that we call cancer. The disease of cancer is a by-product of lifestyle and environmental factors and not of some gene gone awry. Moreover, the aging process does not have to carry an increased risk of cancer. Cancer is avoidable.

In this chapter, we will discuss the factors responsible for cancer, outline what everyone can do to keep it from occurring, and provide information to those who are trying to prevent its recurrence. Finally, we will provide information to those of you undergoing cancer treatment.

Cancer Statistics

Cancer remains the second leading cause of death in North America, surpassed only by heart disease. It is also the main reason people don't make it beyond the average life expectancy. In the year 2002, over 130,000 Canadians and almost 1.3 million Americans were told they had cancer. About 40 percent of the North American population will develop cancer at some point in their lives. Almost 85 percent of all cancers are diagnosed in individuals aged 50 and older.[2]

The four most common types of cancer are breast, prostate, lung, and colon. About one in eight women will develop breast cancer, and the statistic is the same for men with respect to prostate cancer. These two cancers represent the greatest risks for women and men. Cigarette smoking is responsible for 30 percent of all cancer deaths. Avoiding tobacco is a step in the right direction, but let's examine other factors.[3]

Factors in the Development of Cancer

Genetics

The evidence shows that genetic inheritance has very little to do with who gets cancer. In a recent study, 44,778 pairs of twins from Finland, Sweden, and Denmark were surveyed for cancer occurrence. The researchers concluded that inherited genetic factors make only a minor contribution to a person's susceptibility of breast, prostate, and colorectal cancer, while environmental factors make a major contribution to the 28 sites of cancer studied.[4]

Researchers from the American Institute for Cancer Research (AICR) agree with the study's findings. The AICR has maintained all along that cancer is largely preventable if you have a proper diet rich in fruits and vegetables, maintain a healthy weight, exercise regularly, and avoid tobacco. The institute has estimated that 70 percent of all cancers can be avoided if these wise lifestyle choices are taken.

Again, a history of cancer in your family does not mean that you will develop the disease. Your genetic inheritance may show you where your family's health has faltered, but it does not promise you a health future no better than theirs. While the risk of developing a disease can be inherited, diseases are very rarely the result of some pre-programmed genetic process that is independent of other factors. Age-related chronic diseases like cancer are linked to lifestyle. In other words, if you behave like your parents, eat what they ate, deal with stress the way they did, and are exposed to the same environmental factors, yes, then you'll probably get what they got out of life.

Body Weight and Exercise

Cancer rates have proportionately increased as the North American population has become heavier. Women who are obese in their post-menopausal years have a 50 percent greater risk of developing breast cancer than women who maintain ideal body weight. Obese men run a 40 percent greater risk of developing colon cancer than men of ideal weight. Obesity increases the risk of breast, endometrial, cervix, ovarian, and gallbladder cancer for women and colon and prostate cancer for men.[5]

Everyone knows the importance of exercise in disease prevention. Those who say they don't have time for exercise will have to make time for illness in their later years. A lifetime of physical inactivity greatly increases cancer risk for both women and men.[6] Health authorities have consistently recommended that you exercise at least 30 minutes five times weekly.

Stress, Mental Attitude, and Emotional Disposition

There is ample evidence to show that one's approach to life is linked to cancer occurrence. Over a 30-year period, Dr. Caroline B. Thomas collected psychological profiles on incoming medical students at the Johns Hopkins School of Medicine in Baltimore, Maryland. She looked at the way these individuals expressed (or didn't express) emotions and the diseases they tended to develop. Keep in mind that medical students typically endure grueling stress, long hours, lack of sleep and exercise, improper diet, isolation, and psychological abuse—a lifestyle that might well influence how they will cope with things later on in life. This is the doctor's rite of passage.

Generally, medical students are not encouraged to express their feelings, but it was found that the students who kept things bottled up were more likely than the others to develop fatal cancers of all types in later years.[7] On the other hand, the students who didn't suppress their feelings but instead exhibited excessive hostility had a fourfold greater risk of developing heart disease.[8] These two emotional dispositions, suppression and hostility, are common throughout society. Is it any wonder, then, that heart disease and cancer are so prevalent these days? There is more.

One's state of mind can affect immune status. It has been shown that shortly after men lose their wives to breast cancer, their immune function is markedly affected. Although the two main cells of the immune system (the T and B lymphocytes) didn't decrease in number, they stopped working for the entire time the men were grieving.[9] Other studies have also suggested that a psychological state of loss has a negative effect on immune status.[10]

Prolonged feelings of loneliness can also depress immune function. Seventy-six first-year medical students at Ohio State University were given extensive psychological tests. Those with the highest loneliness and stress scores had the lowest levels of natural killer (NK) cells, while those with the lowest scores of loneliness had the highest levels of NK cells.[11] NK cells are the body's warrior cells that search for and destroy rogue cancer cells.

The feeling of being connected, of belonging, is very important for the immune function. In another study, about 7,000 healthy adults from Alameda County, California, were examined to determine whether there was a relationship between social isolation and cancer occurrence. Women who felt lonely despite having many social contacts were 2.4 times more likely to develop and die from hormone-dependent cancers (breast, ovarian, and uterine). Women who felt lonely and had few social contacts were 5 times more likely to develop and die from these cancers. For men, there was no observable relationship between a lack of strong social ties and cancer occurrence. However, socially isolated men who developed cancer tended to die much sooner than expected.[12]

While cancer has many causes, prolonged stress, lack of mental and emotional harmony, isolation, and loneliness have a lot to do with cancer development.

Diet

The ongoing scrutiny of diet has revealed definite links between what we eat and our risk of developing cancer. In 1997 the American Institute for Cancer Research published a report on the results of more than 4,500 studies on diet and cancer occurrence. This report concluded that diets that downplay meat and dairy and focus on vegetables, fruits, whole grains, and beans significantly decrease the risk of cancer.[13]

At least 40 micronutrients (these would include vitamins and minerals) are required in the human diet, and a frequently asked question is, Do micronutrient deficiencies in today's diets explain the high cancer rates? According to researchers, a deficiency in at least eight micronutrients (vitamins C, E, B6, B12, folic acid, niacin, iron, and zinc) exposes DNA to extensive damage, similar to that caused by radiation and chemical exposure. DNA controls cellular division, and when it accrues extensive damage, cancer is a likely consequence. The percentage of the U.S. population deficient in these micronutrients ranges from 2 to 20+ percent.[14]

Keep in mind that a *deficiency* means that you would be taking in less than 50 percent of the RDA (recommended daily allowance). The above percentages would be even greater if the people who don't get 100 percent of the RDA were included. Furthermore, many health advocates believe that many of those who meet the RDA receive insufficient amounts of micronutrients for their particular needs.[15]

Interestingly, evidence suggests that low levels of selenium in the soil of various areas of the world correlate with higher rates of cancer. Selenium bolsters immune function and protects against DNA damage caused by free radicals. Many scientists have concluded that a daily supplemental dose of 200 micrograms of selenium helps to prevent cancer. This dose greatly exceeds the RDA and cannot be easily obtained from dietary sources alone. As with vitamins E and C, the door has opened for selenium supplementation in cancer prevention.[16]

More than 200 epidemiological studies have shown that low fruit and vegetable intake translates into higher rates of cancer. The quarter of the U.S. population that eats the least amount of fruits and vegetables has about twice the incidence of cancer as the quarter of the population that eats the greatest amount of nutrient-dense foods. About 75 percent of American children, adolescents, and adults don't eat the recommended minimum amount of five servings of fruits and vegetables. Sadly, the fruits and vegetables favored by North Americans are iceberg lettuce, french fries, tomatoes, and orange juice. These foods are low in micronutrients and fiber, high in sugar, and, in the case of french fries, high in trans fatty acids. And only a fraction of the 4,000 phytochemicals are consumed with this typical diet. This is unfortunate, since high blood levels of phytochemicals, particularly the carotenoids obtained from carrots and cruciferous and green leafy vegetables, help prevent cancer.[17]

Caloric intake, the type and amount of fat, protein, and carbohydrates in the diet, and fiber intake also influence cancer rates. The general consensus among cancer researchers is that a diet high in calories and saturated fat and low in fiber increases the risk of cancer.[18] On average, North Americans consume only about 12 grams of fiber daily. The U.S. National Cancer Institute recommends a minimum of 25 grams and suggests, on the basis of worldwide population studies, that 35–40 grams of fiber daily is optimal to prevent cancer.[19]

The fatty acid ratio (omega-6 to omega-3) in the typical North American diet falls in the range of 15:1 to 20:1, ratios believed to be responsible for high cancer rates. It has been shown that a ratio of 4:1 translates into very low cancer rates. The diet on the Greek island of Crete, for example, has a good balance of fatty acids and is abundant in fruits, vegetables, nuts, seeds, whole grains, fiber, fish, olive oil, vitamins C and E, selenium, and plant antioxidants, and Cretans have a very low risk of developing cancer. This dietary pattern is popularly known as the Mediterranean diet.[20]

The Biological Terrain of Cancer

Just as sugar consumption has skyrocketed in North America over the last 150 years, so too has the incidence of cancer. The consumption of refined grains has also risen proportionately. Studies show that increasing your consumption of refined grains (breads, pasta, baked goods, rice) can double your risk of cancer.[21]

An intake of too many calories (especially from carbohydrates and refined white flour and sugar) and physical inactivity can lead to insulin resistance. Some form of insulin resistance is an inevitable age-related phenomenon, created by hyperinsulinemia (high blood levels of insulin). However, does insulin resistance and hyperinsulinemia create the biochemical fertility required by cancer for its growth? According to one study, the answer is yes. Its findings suggest that hyperinsulinemia and insulin resistance increase the risk not only of obesity, diabetes, and heart disease but also of cancer. Chronically elevated insulin levels stimulate the cells of the body to divide rapidly before they need to. A high rate of cell division exposes the cells to mutations that can lead to cancerous growths.[22]

Insulin resistance means that sugar accumulates in the blood. Excessive blood sugar promotes the growth of systemic fungus, and according to one study, chronic fungal infections are capable of turning normal cells into cancerous ones. Indeed, a link might be drawn between cancer and persistent fungal infections because of the high incidence of both in North America.[23]

Environmental Toxicity

Our environment is strewn with many pitfalls. Why, for example, are fungal infections so common? The answer lies in the overuse of antibiotics. Antibiotics destroy the beneficial bacteria that keep harmful bacteria in check. The common fungus *Candida albicans*, for instance, normally present in low numbers, is allowed to proliferate and over a long period can cause problems for the immune system.

Over 100,000 man-made chemicals circulate throughout our environment, with hundreds added every year. The list of known and suspected carcinogens continues to grow. We accrue these ubiquitous toxins in our body tissues. And as our environment becomes increasingly polluted, the risk of cancer increases exponentially. As we damage the environment, we damage ourselves.

Carcinogens

If you eat a lot of barbecued, smoked, and otherwise adulterated meat, your cancer risk increases. The compounds formed from barbecuing meat and the preservatives and flavoring agents added to other meats are known carcinogens. Women who consistently eat well-done steak, hamburgers, and bacon have a 4.62 times greater risk of getting breast cancer than women who don't have this diet.[24] Marinating meat for at least two hours before cooking and then slow-roasting it prevents the formation of carcinogens. Marinades that contain olive oil, vinegar, garlic, mustard, lemon juice, rosemary, oregano, and curcumin have been shown to be ideal.[25]

It's worth the extra cost to select hormone-free chicken and beef. Some experts are convinced that North American men have the highest rates of prostate cancer in the world because the meat they consume is contaminated with growth hormones. In the United States, more than a dozen different growth hormones are used to fatten cattle. These hormones mimic estrogen, and excessive estrogen stimulation in men is a key factor in the development of prostate cancer.[26] Canadians are at equal risk because some of the U.S. beef makes its way into Canada.

Women may want to rethink hormone replacement therapy (HRT) for the treatment of menopause. According to the U.S. National Institute of Environmental Health Services, conjugated estrogens (i.e., the type of estrogens prescribed for HRT in menopausal women) are carcinogenic.[27] There is evidence to show that the longer women take conjugated estrogens, the more significant their risk of breast cancer compared with that of women who never took HRT in their menopausal years. Adding synthetic progestins to conjugated estrogens does not reduce the cancer risk. Many researchers have stated that HRT may be inappropriate, especially for women who have a family history of breast cancer.[28]

Cancer Prevention

While cancer has numerous causes, no one needs to feel defeated, even if there is a history of cancer in the family. As noted earlier, cancer is not genetically programmed; nor is it a process that is switched on and develops overnight. Cancer is a disease process that may take decades to develop. It does not spring up in a day.

The body's ability to protect itself against cancer hinges upon some of the body's well-known functions—specifically, its ability to destroy infectious microbes, eliminate metabolic waste and environmental toxins, and repair cellular damage. The fact that almost half of all cancers are in hormone-sensitive tissues suggests that there is a need for greater hormonal control. Furthermore, 20 percent of all cancers occur in the digestive system, confirming that diet is hugely significant in cancer prevention. Therapies designed to support these areas would most assuredly help. Let's look at some specific things you can do to prevent cancer.

1. Don't smoke, and avoid secondhand smoke, alcohol, and illicit drugs. It's best to avoid caffeinated beverages. If you drink coffee, have no more than 16 ounces daily. Avoid pesticide- and chemical-laden coffee.

2. Exercise regularly. Incorporate a variety of exercises that include deep breathing, relaxation techniques, stretching, strength training, and a cardiovascular workout.

3. Adopt a healthy lifestyle, and that includes getting adequate sleep, rest, and relaxation. Develop strategies to manage stress effectively. Be mentally positive and emotionally balanced. Make sure your spiritual needs are met. Develop close, loving, and supportive relationships.

4. Maintain your ideal body weight.

5. Eat a whole-foods, plant-based diet. Eat at least five servings of a variety of fresh fruits and vegetables daily. Eat a variety of whole grains, fresh raw nuts and seeds, and beans. Make sure your diet includes at least 25 grams of fiber daily. Reduce saturated fat intake; no more than 25 percent of your total daily calories should come from fat. Eat cancer-fighting foods, herbs, and spices, such as garlic, ginger, cayenne, rosemary, oregano, and curcumin. Avoid high-calorie, low-nutrient foods that are high in refined carbohydrates, trans fatty acids, food additives, and dyes (e.g., snack foods, baked goods, junk foods, and fast foods). Avoid barbecued, charred, or well-done blackened meat; marinated, slow-roasted meat is best. Choose certified organic (i.e., hormone-free, antibiotic-free, pesticide-free, quality-fed and -raised) beef, chicken, and eggs high in omega-3 fatty acids. To get more omega-3 fatty acids, eat fish twice a week and add flaxseed to your diet. Eat soy-protein foods. Eat three well-balanced meals at regular times of the day, and don't skip meals.

6. Drink at least six 8-ounce glasses of pure water daily. Make water your beverage of choice. Drink at least one cup of quality green tea daily. If you like fruit and vegetable juices, use a juicer or squeezer so that they're fresh.

7. Be environmentally conscious. After all, if you pollute your environment, you pollute your own body. Recycle as much as possible. Choose chemical-free, carcinogen-free, biodegradable household cleaning agents and health and beauty products. Avoid using chemical pesticides and fertilizers on your lawn and garden; there are safer alternatives. Before you eat from your garden, have the soil inspected. Make sure the air in your home is properly filtered; keep it free of mold, mildew, and other germs. The same goes for your workplace. Use sunscreen when you're exposed to sunlight for prolonged periods. Avoid unnecessary X-rays and other forms of electromagnetic radiation.

8. See your doctor yearly for a thorough health examination. Discuss with your doctor what you can do to prevent cancer. Report to him or her major changes in bowel and bladder function, a persistent cough, sore throat, or hoarseness, chronic swollen glands, difficulty swallowing or ingesting food, lumps in breasts or testicles, wounds or sores that are slow to heal, unusual bleeding, and changes in warts, moles, or other growths on the skin, as these may be signs of cancer.

9. Develop a sensible and well-balanced nutritional supplement program in which quality, purity, and safety are emphasized. Take a high-potency multiple vitamin and mineral supplement. Make sure you get 200–400 micrograms of selenium, 400–800 IUs of vitamin E (natural mixed tocopherols), and 500–5,000 milligrams of vitamin C. Make sure your diet has a good balance of omega-6 and omega-3 fatty acids; you can do this by taking 2 tablespoons of Udo's Ultimate Oil Blend daily. If you find it difficult to get the minimum daily requirement of 25 grams of fiber from your diet, consider supplemental powders that come in both soluble and insoluble forms. Consider taking adaptogenic phytomedicines; these essentially act as tonics, protecting the body from a variety of stress-induced damage.

10. Detoxify and cleanse your body at least twice a year (refer to Chapter 9). After cleansing, adjust your basic nutritional supplement program in order to give your body support where it is needed most. Make sure that your digestive, immune, and nervous systems are functioning optimally; all other systems in your body are dependent on the proper functioning of these three (refer to chapters 9, 11, and 17, respectively).

Preventing the Recurrence of Cancer

Many people who have had cancer look at life and see new opportunities. For them it's a chance to do things differently, to eat differently, to live differently, and to tend to things long neglected. Indeed, some see their illness as a time to deal with the emotional trauma of their lives and find resolution. Certainly, people should conquer a fear of their cancer returning in order to move forward in good health.

Despite their success rate, cancer treatments such as surgery, radiation, drug therapy, and chemotherapy are traumatic for the body. For instance, radiation and chemotherapy are targeted to kill all rapidly dividing cancerous cells, but because the cells of the gut are also rapidly dividing, renewing the tissues of the gut every seven days, radiation and especially chemotherapy cause the gut to shrink or atrophy. Refer back to Chapter 10 to see how you can nourish the gut and restore its function. The immune system and overall health are dependent on a well-functioning gut.

Medicinal Mushrooms

While there are numerous medicinal mushrooms and natural plant compounds, we will mention just one. In over 400 trials, *Coriolus versicolor,* commonly known as turkey tail or cloud mushroom, has been confirmed to improve overall health. It has also been shown to build immune function and improve recovery when given before or after surgery to patients with gastric, colorectal, lung, and breast cancer. Equally important, compared with cancer patients who didn't take *Coriolus versicolor,* those who did remained in remission and disease free for significantly longer periods and their survival rates beyond five years were much higher. *Coriolus versicolor* modifies all aspects of immune function, improves liver health, helps to rebuild the gut, controls inflammation, and deals with the toxicity generated by chemotherapy. Organika's Coriolus Versicolor (available under the traditional name, Yun Zhi) is made to exacting standards and contains the therapeutic compounds that provide the multiple benefits mentioned above.[29] (See Appendix 7.1.)

Treating Cancer

Throughout most of the world, biological and nutritional therapies are employed alongside medical treatment to improve recovery and survival rates for cancer patients. However, the majority of oncologists in North America discourage their cancer patients from taking natural products and nutritional supplements, especially antioxidants. The reason often cited is that such things interfere with radiation and chemotherapy treatment. Is this really true?

If we ask whether there exists any evidence showing that nutritional supplements or natural products are of benefit to cancer patients undergoing radiation or chemotherapy, we find that the answer is yes. Over the last 30 years, hundreds of scientific studies have shown that patients experience multiple benefits from nutritional supplements given in conjunction with chemotherapy and radiation. These benefits include the prevention of weight loss, nausea and vomiting, diarrhea, immune system depression, and secondary infection. Improvements in energy levels, well-being, sleep, digestion, and elimination have also been reported. Furthermore, enhancement of—not interference with—chemotherapy has been demonstrated; supplements have been shown to reduce the toxicity of chemotherapy, and with their use, more aggressive chemotherapy treatments can be administered without delay and without complications. Most important, cancer patients who use nutritional and natural supplements under medical supervision typically recover more quickly and survive longer than those patients who do not.[30]

Conclusion

Which is more critical in the development of cancer, genes or the environment? It should be clear to you by now that the likelihood of your developing cancer has much more to do with your lifestyle, the foods you eat, and the environment around you than with the genes you've inherited. Your approach to life, your psychological and emotional tendencies, and the quality of your relationships also have a tremendous impact on your susceptibility to cancer.

The aging of the North American population does not explain today's high cancer rates; nor does genetic inheritance. Cancer is preventable, and so are all other age-related diseases. To avoid what have been considered the inevitable afflictions of aging, you must pull together all the therapeutic aspects outlined in this chapter and throughout the book. In doing so, you will have the health you need to pursue a happy life.

CONCLUSION

We hope that the 20 chapters of this book will have convinced you, first and foremost, that the natural process of aging doesn't inevitably include disease and disability. Medical science has succeeded in identifying common features that influence the rate of aging and all age-related diseases. Our understanding of aging is now at the level of what happens inside the cells of the body. Aging can no longer be viewed as a series of biochemical reactions controlled solely by genetic inheritance.

While it is true that genetic inheritance determines many of your characteristics, the quality and length of your life are influenced by a variety of factors that interact with your genes. An inadequate diet, unhealthy environmental conditions, and a demanding lifestyle—mentally, physically, and emotionally—are read as stress by everyone's genes. You shouldn't worry so much about what you've inherited from your parents; instead you should be concerned about how much stress your genes can take before giving way to disease and rapid aging. Inside everyone lies the genetic potential for good health. Your health fate is contingent upon your surroundings, your diet, and the way you deal with stress.

Stress is a theme that runs throughout this book. This should not be surprising, as it is at the root of almost all chronic degenerative diseases. The majority of individuals will spend half of their remaining years with declining health and disease, indications that their stress has not been managed effectively. Stress is essential to life, and if you make the right choices, it can promote physical, psychological, and spiritual growth.

Many people reach the age of 100 with all aspects of their health intact. Their successful aging shows that health can be synonymous with longevity. In fact, there's a good deal of interest in the idea that we have enough genetic material in us to live for 120 to 140 years. Unfortunately, no therapies have actually gotten anybody that distance. Still, at one time the moon was out of reach. We don't know whether such long lives will eventually be available to everyone, but we do know that healthy aging can be achieved by virtually all of us, since age-related diseases are largely avoidable.

The prevention formulas provided in these pages can't be followed for just a few weeks and then discarded. If you are seeking enduring health and vitality, you must follow the recommendations on an ongoing basis. Even those with chronic diseases can reap benefits. To ensure progress, keep this book handy and refer to it every step of the way.

Recent discoveries in the nutritional sciences have provided a wealth of plant-derived supplements and medicines that can help you maximize your functional health span. They have opened new frontiers in conquering disease and optimizing health. These science-based products, however, should be incorporated into the health programs presented in this book. Taken alone, they are of little value.

In our vision of the future, people will no longer suffer from the physical limitations associated with aging. They will live longer lives, and they will have the necessary health and vigor to find fulfillment and happiness. You can begin this journey by adopting a healthy lifestyle right now and sticking with it. *Breaking the Age Barrier* is the beginning of a better health future for you. Cheers!

APPENDICES

APPENDIX 2.1
BENEFITS OF PHYTOCHEMICALS

PLANT COMPOUNDS	FOOD SOURCE	EFFECTS
Anthocyanosides	Bilberry, blueberries	Strengthen capillaries; improve night vision; support light/dark adaptation; protect retina; protect against eye strain and fatigue, macular degeneration, glaucoma, cataracts, and varicose veins
Carotenes (beta carotene)	Carrots and numerous fruits and vegetables	Protect against cancer, heart disease; improve immune function
Curcuminoids	Turmeric root	Lower cholesterol; improve circulation, immune, and digestive function; control inflammation; protect against heart disease and cancer
D-glucarate, indole-3-carbinol (I3C), sulforaphanes	Apples, oranges, grapefruit, broccoli, Brussels sprouts, cabbage, cauliflower, kale	Improve detoxification; protect against cancer; balance hormones
Gingerols	Ginger	Control inflammation and infections; improve circulation, digestion, and liver and gallbladder function
Lutein	Tomatoes, spinach, kale, and other dark-green leafy vegetables	Supports eye health; protects against cancer
Lycopene	Tomatoes, watermelon	Protects against heart disease and prostate and pancreatic cancer
Polyphenols	Green tea	Lower cholesterol; protect against heart disease and cancer; improve detoxification
Sulfur compounds	Garlic	Stimulate immune system; direct antimicrobial effects to control infectious diseases; protect against cancer and heart disease; control cholesterol and blood sugar and pressure; improve circulation; bind heavy metals out of system

APPENDIX 4.1
RECORDING YOUR BIOMARKERS

Height: _____

Weight: _____

Body mass index (BMI): _____

Percentage body fat: _____

Muscle mass: _____

Bone density: _____

Blood pressure: _____

Heartbeats per minute: _____

Total cholesterol to HDL cholesterol ratio: _____

Blood glucose (fasting) or glucose-tolerance test: _____

Insulin levels (fasting): _____

Homocysteine levels: _____

Thyroid function test: _____

Liver function test: _____

Complete blood counts (to rule out anemia or immune deficiencies): _____

Prostate-specific antigen (PSA) and prostate examination: _____

Breast examination and mammography: _____

Eye examination: _____

Hearing examination: _____

APPENDIX 4.2
BIOLOGICAL AGE QUESTIONNAIRE

Biological age is a measure of your inner health, which is influenced by your genetics and your lifestyle choices. Biological age is an effective indicator of your "true" age because it measures how well you are taking care of your body by rating the damage your body has undergone in its lifetime.

This questionnaire provides an inner profile by measuring the extent of internal damage your body has accumulated. To achieve an accurate measure of your biological age, it is important to answer the questions as accurately and honestly as possible. The Biological Age Questionnaire is easy to follow and can be completed at your convenience.

Section A – Chronological Age

1. What is your current age (in years)?
    _____ **Total Score (Section A)**

Section B – Dietary Choices

2. How frequently do you eat fried, broiled, or barbecued foods?
    Often = 4
    Once a day = 3
    Few times per week = 2
    Once a week = 1
    Almost never = –2

3. How often do you consume nutritional oils (not fried or heated)? (example: flaxseed oil)
    Never = 2
    Once a week = 1
    Once a day = 0
    2+ times per day = –1

4. How many servings of fruit or vegetables do you consume? (1 serving = 1 cup)
    Almost never = 3
    Few times per week = 2
    One per day = 1
    3 per day = –1
    5+ per day = –2

5. How often do you consume whole grains and/or natural fiber? (example: whole wheat, psyllium, brown or wild rice)
    Almost never = 3
    Once a week = 2
    Few times per week = 1
    Often = –2

6. How many glasses of water do you consume daily? (water does not include coffee, black tea, soda, alcohol)
    Almost never = 3
    One per day = 2
    4 per day = 1
    8 per day = 0
    10+ per day = –2

7. Do you consume sugar, soda, white flour, or other processed foods? (example: canned foods, fast food, TV dinners, foods with preservatives added)
3+ times per day = 3
Once a day = 2
Few times per week = 1
Almost never = −1

8. How many alcoholic drinks do you consume per week?
12+ per week = 3
8 per week = 2
4 per week = 1
2 per week = 0
Almost never = −1

9. How often do you add salt to your food?
All food = 3
Daily = 2
Few times per week = 1
Once a month = 0
Almost never = −1
_____Total Score (Section B)

Section C – Dietary Supplementation

10. Do you take a multivitamin?
Almost never = 2
Once a week = 1
Few times per week = 0
Daily = −1

11. Do you take antioxidants? (example: grape seed extract, selenium)
Almost never = 3
Once a week = 2
Few times per week = 1
Daily = −2
_____Total Score (Section C)

Section D – Daily Activities

12. Do you exercise (30 or more minutes of continuous activity)?
Almost never = 3
Once a week = 2
3 times per week = −2
5+ times per week = −3

13. When you exercise, do you do so for more than 2 hours? (If you do not exercise, please put "0" as your answer.)
Most times = 4
50% of the time = 2
Almost never = 0

14. Do you sleep well and awake rested?
Almost never = 3
Sometimes = 2
Usually = 0
Always = −1

15. How often do you have normal bowel movements?
Once a week = 4
Every 4 days = 3
Every second day = 2
Daily = 0
2+ times per day = −2
_____ Total Score (Section D)

Section E – Medical History

16. Is there a history of the following conditions in your family? (cancer, diabetes, heart disease, depression, obesity, liver disease, high cholesterol, high blood pressure)
2 or more = 1
One = 0
None = −1

17. Have you ever had any of the following conditions? (cancer, diabetes, heart disease, depression, obesity, liver disease, high cholesterol, high blood pressure)
2 or more = 3
One = 2
None = –2

18. How frequently do you experience the following conditions? (headache, fever, sore throat, muscle aches [not exercise induced], colds or flu, rash, swelling)
Once a day = 3
Once a week = 2
Once a month = 0
Almost never = –1

19. Have you ever been exposed to heavy metals or toxic substances? (examples: mechanics, hair dressers, nail technicians, etc.)
Daily = 4
Weekly = 3
Monthly = 2
Almost never = 0

20. Have you ever been exposed to heavy metals via dental work or fillings? (example: mercury fillings or other metal fillings)
3+ fillings = 4
2 fillings = 3
1 filling = 2
Never = 0
_____ Total Score (Section E)

Section F – Stress

21. How many full meals do you eat per day? (a snack is not a full meal)
Never = 3
4+ per day = 3
3 per day = 0
2 per day = 1
One per day = 2

22. At work or at home, how often are you in front of electronic equipment? (example: computers, television, live cameras, electrical wires)
8+ hours per day = 3
6+ hours per day = 2
Few hours per day = 1
Almost never = 0

23. How often are you exposed to cigarette smoke (direct or second-hand)?
All day = 4
Few times a day = 3
Few times per week = 1
Almost never = –1

24. Do you use recreational or street drugs?
2+ times per day = 4
Once a day = 3
Once a week = 2
Once a month = 1
Never = 0

25. Do you drive in heavy traffic?
For a living = 3
Daily (3+ hours) = 2
Daily (1–2 hours) = 1
Almost never = –1

26. At work and/or home, do you experience stress?
Very high = 4
High = 3
Moderate = 2
Slight = 1
Almost none = –2
_____ Total Score (Section F)

Calculating Your Biological Age

Add the scores from the following sections together to calculate your biological age:

Section A – Chronological Age _____

Section B – Dietary Choices _____

Section C – Dietary Supplementation ___

Section D – Daily Activities _____

Section E – Medical History _____

Section F – Stress _____

Total Score _____

Your Biological Age _____

Evaluating the Results:

If your biological age is:

A. Minus 11 years or greater (biological age eleven or more years less than your chronological age)

   General health picture is excellent. The right choices are being made to ensure your continued health.

B. Minus 1–10 years (biological age is one to ten years less than your chronological age)

   General health picture is very good. Focus on maintaining your healthy lifestyle choices, diet, exercise, and stress management.

C. Biological age is the same as your chronological age

   General health picture is good. However, changes are required to achieve optimal health and maximize energy levels. Proper dietary choices are vital for improved health.

D. 1–10 years plus (biological age one to ten years greater than your chronological age)

   General health picture is fair. However, following the same lifestyle will cause biological age to rise and heighten the risk of serious health problems. Improved dietary choices are required to avoid future health risks.

E. 11–20 years plus (biological age eleven to twenty years greater than your chronological age)

   General health picture is average, as this is the most common health picture, with a moderate risk of health complications in the next five years. Energy and mobility are starting to decline and will continue to do so. Dietary changes are essential for improving overall health.

F. 21 years plus (biological age twenty-one or more years greater than your chronological age)

   A chronic degenerative health picture, with a high risk of developing serious health complications. Energy and mobility will seriously decline in the next few years (if they have not already). Dietary and lifestyle changes are essential for improving overall health. Stress must be reduced. Physical activity is a great way to reduce stress while at the same time improving health and increasing energy.

Reprinted with permission from Flora Manufacturing & Distributing, Ltd., Burnaby, BC, Canada.

APPENDIX 7.1
DIRECTORY OF SUPPLEMENT MANUFACTURERS

Advanced Orthomolecular Research (AOR)
4101 19th Street NE
Bay #9
Calgary, AB
T2E 6X8
(403) 250-9997
(800) 387-0177

Description: AOR manufactures and distributes high-quality, research-based natural products. They carry a comprehensive line of novel compounds, such as Prostaphil-2™, R(+)-Lipoic Acid, Citocline, Methyl Cobalamine, Indole-3-Carbinol (I3C), Phosphatidyl-choline (PC), and Phosphatidyl-Serine (PS), for specific therapeutic uses.

Ehn
317 Adelaide Street West
Suite 501
Toronto, ON
M5V 1P9
(416) 977-8765
(416) 977-4184 (fax)
Website: www.greenspluscanada.com

Description: Ehn is the manufacturer and developer of high-quality nutritional supplements such as greens+™, A·G·E inhibitors™, and protect™. Their products and programs have been designed to address many of the changes seen in aging and age-related diseases. They are to be used as part of an overall health-promoting whole-foods diet and lifestyle.

Enzymatic Therapy
2696 Nookta Street
Vancouver, BC
V5N 3N5
(604) 421-0777
(604) 421-0557 (fax)
(800) 665-3414
Website: www.enzymaticcanada.com

Description: Enzymatic Therapy is known for its dedication to creating an innovative line of quality health supplements. Their line includes Remifemin, DGL, Standardized Extracts, Phytosomes, Esberitox, and IP-6.

Flora
7400 Fraser Park Drive
Burnaby, BC
V5J 5B9
(604) 436-6000
(604) 436-6060 (fax)
(888) 436-6697
Website: www.florahealth.com

Description: Flora is one of North America's premier manufacturers and distributors of natural health products. They manufacture and distribute Udo's Ultimate Oil Blend®, an organic and unrefined blend of plant-based oils that provides a balanced intake of omega-6 and omega-3 fatty acids.

Inno-Vite Inc.
97 Saramia Crescent
Concord, ON
L4K 4P7
(905) 761-5121
(905) 761-1453 (fax)
(800) 387-9111

Description: Since 1983, Inno-Vite has provided Canadians with unique, high-quality natural products that adhere to strict quality control and third-party lab testing. The Inno-Vite brand leads in cardiovascular natural remedies with Formula H.H. and Co-enzyme Q10 M.R.B. (Maximum Relative Bio-Availability) Q-GelR; it also leads in candidiasis recovery with the Yeast BusterT program, including KolorexR. Inno-Vite also brings you therapeutic DDSR Acidophilus, Flora-GloR Lutein, Starch Stopper Phase 2, and more.

The Institute for Functional Medicine
Gig Harbor Corporate Center
4411 Point Fosdick Drive NW
Gig Harbor, WA
(253) 858-4724
(800) 228-0622
Website: www.functionalmedicine.org

Description: IFM is a non-profit organization that educates health-care practitioners worldwide on the use of functional foods and biological medicines in improving health outcomes. Over its more than 10-year history, the institute's many evidence-based articles have contributed to the better health and well-being of thousands of patients. This organization can provide referrals to well-trained health-care practitioners who practice functional medicine in your area.

Jamieson Laboratories Ltd.
4025 Rhodes Drive
Windsor, ON
N8W 5B5
(519) 974-8482
(519) 974-4742 (fax)
(800) 265-5053
Website: www.jamiesonvitamins.com

Description: Jamieson Labs is a manufacturer, formulator, and marketer of an extensive line of quality nutritional supplements, including vitamins, minerals, and herbs. They have a state-of-the-art research laboratory and manufacturing facility that produces products for 26 countries.

Metagenics, Canada
851 Rangeview Road
Mississauga, ON
L5E 1H1
(905) 891-1300
(800) 268-6200

Metagenics, USA
100 Avenida La Pata
San Clemente, CA 92673
(949) 366-0818
(800) 692-9400
Website: www.metagenics.com

Description: Metagenics was founded almost 20 years ago with the goal of optimizing "genetic potential through nutrition." Its expert team of research scientists develops cutting-edge nutritional formulas to improve health outcomes. Many of Metagenics' products have received U.S. patents. UltraInflamX™ (UltraInflavogen in Canada), UltraClear PLUS®, Ulcinex™, and Endefen™ are just a few of its products.

Natural Factors Nutritional Products
1350 United Blvd.
Coquitlam, BC
V3K 6Y7
(604) 420-4229
(604) 420-0772 (fax)
(800) 663-8900
Website: www.naturalfactors.com

Description: Natural Factors manufactures an extensive line of supplements, including vitamins, minerals, and herbs. This company is committed to researching and developing quality supplements to enhance the well-being of its customers. Its products are available in Canada and the United States.

Organika® Health Products, Inc.
11871 Hammersmith Way
Richmond, BC
V7A 5E5
(604) 277-3302
(604) 277-3352 (fax)
Website: www.organika.com

Description: Organika® is a Canadian company that manufactures and distributes an extensive line of high-quality nutritional supplements and phytomedicines. Organika was the first company to introduce to Canadian consumers GLS 500® Sodium Free Glucosamine Sulfate, a product that has now been available for almost 10 years. Full Spectrum Plant Enzymes®, Yun Zhi Mushroom Extract Coriolus Versicolor, and Cordyceps Mushroom Extract are also manufactured and distributed by Organika.

PanGeo Health Brands, Inc.
2180 Dunwin Drive
Units 2 and 3
Mississauga, ON
L5L 5M8
(905) 828-3530
(905) 828-3531 (fax)
Website: www.questvitamins.com

Description: PanGeo distributes and manufactures Quest Vitamins, a Canadian company that has been providing consumers with premium-quality and research-based nutritional products since 1976. Some of the nutritional formulas by Quest are Ginsana®, Ginkoba®, EstroLogic™, Kyolic Aged Garlic Extract™, OsteoLogic™, and TrimFit™.

Prairie Naturals®

1772 Broadway Street

Suite 106-B

Port Coquitlam, BC

V3C 2M8

(604) 941-4950

(604) 941-4974 (fax)

(800) 931-4247

Website: www.prairienaturals.com

Description: Prairie Naturals®, a Canadian company, manufactures and distributes hypoallergenic nutritional supplements that are available in easy-to-take capsules, powder, and liquid form. Prairie Naturals distributes Multi-Force and ReCleanse™.

Purity Life Health Products

6 Commerce Crescent

Acton, ON

L7J 2X3

(519) 853-3511

(519) 853-4660 (fax)

(800) 265-2615

Website: www.puritylife.com

Description: Purity Life is Canada's largest independent distributor of natural health-care products, including nutritional supplements and body-care products. Purity Life is committed to "empowering people to create well-being in their lives." They are the exclusive distributors for the research-based immune formula Moducare®.

SISU Enterprises Co., Inc.

104-A – 3430 Brighton Avenue

Burnaby, BC

V5A 3H4

(604) 420-6610

(604) 420-6640 (fax)

(800) 663-4163

Website: www.sisuhealth.com

Description: Using the highest quality-control standards and technology, SISU manufactures and distributes an innovative line of natural health products.

Solgar Vitamin and Herb

6505 Edwards Blvd.

Mississauga, ON

L5T 2V2

(905) 564-1154

(905) 507-5524 (fax)

Website: www.solgar.com

Description: Since 1947, Solgar Vitamin and Herb has been committed to the total health and well-being of consumers worldwide. They distribute an extensive line of supplements, including vitamins, minerals, herbs, and food supplements, in Canada and the United States.

Swiss Herbal Remedies Ltd.

35 Leek Crescent

Richmond Hill, ON

L4B 4C3

(905) 886-9500

(905) 886-5434 (fax)

(800) 268-9879

Website: www.swissherbal.ca

Description: Swiss Herbal provides an extensive line of premium-quality natural-source vitamins, minerals, and herbal supplements, including Cran-Max® and Natural HRT™. All their products are tested for quality, purity, and stability.

Webber Naturals

Unit# 103–3686 Bonneville Place

Burnaby, BC

V3N 4T6

(604) 422 2800

(604) 422-2802 fax

(800) 430-7898

Website: www.wnpharmaceuticals.com

Webber Naturals carries a complete line of natural health products based on years of dedicated research. They select only the purest, highest quality ingredients that meet pharmaceutical standards in product formulation. All of their products are guaranteed for quality, purity, stability, and potency, such as Vitamin E Pure, EchinaMax®, MenoNaturals (Black Cohosh Extract), Saw Palmetto Extract, and MetaSlim™ weight loss products.

APPENDIX 7.2
THE MODIFIED ELIMINATION DIET

An Introductory Word

The following dietary program is designed to remove foods from your diet that are commonly associated with allergies, intolerances, and/or sensitivities. Its focus is on the amount, type, and quality of protein, carbohydrates, fat, and fiber you consume. In general, this food plan provides greater amounts of nutrients than most other diets, as it emphasizes fresh, whole, and organic (when feasible) foods.

Elimination diets have been used therapeutically since the 1920s to solve complex medical problems and improve overall health. They have helped people with environmental allergies, chronic fatigue, chronic inflammatory disorders (e.g., arthritis, asthma, and migraines), frequent headaches, unexplained muscle and joint pain, skin rashes, and gastrointestinal disorders. Their applications are diverse, but they share the same goal of promoting overall health and well-being.

On the basis of clinical observation, many practitioners believe that elimination diets help to optimize gastrointestinal and immune function, regulate blood sugar, control chronic inflammation, and improve the body's ability to eliminate toxins.

The Modified Elimination Diet presented here is not nearly as restrictive as the elimination diets that were used long ago. You won't have to count your calories or feel that you're being starved. Should you decide to follow this diet, there are a number of points to keep in mind:

- Stick with the diet for at least one month.
- Carefully read the guidelines below about what foods are allowed.
- If you have known severe reactions to some of the recommended foods, do not eat them.
- Construct a weekly meal planner that lists the foods you will eat for breakfast, lunch, dinner, and snacks (these foods must among the "allowable" foods described below).
- Stock your cupboards and refrigerator with these foods so that they'll be available to you.
- If you eat out at restaurants, plan ahead and make sure their menus include your allowable foods. Most places can easily accommodate special requests—just ask.
- Refer to your meal planner daily to make sure that you are adhering to the diet.
- Revise your meal planner weekly to get a variety of foods; a varied diet is better for you and will keep you from getting bored with the diet.

- Try to be both organized and creative; you'll find that it's not hard to prepare delicious and convenient meals. You can draw on countless books and websites for recipes.

- The diet may be a radical departure from your usual fare, so be aware that you may have some initial unpleasant experiences—food cravings, body aches, fatigue, digestive disturbances (gas and bloating), and changes in bowel and urinary habits. These "withdrawal symptoms" occur within the first week. They are over quickly, so persevere!

- Keep a daily journal of what you are eating and how you are feeling. At the end of 30 days, most people report mental clarity, sustainable energy levels, better sleep, less physical pain, improved digestion and elimination, and fewer "junk food" cravings.

- After the 30 days, reintroduce one food item each week and take note of its effect on your health. In this way, you will be able to identify the variety of foods that help your body function optimally.

- *If you have a severe illness, take prescription medicines, or are already on a special therapeutic diet, get clearance from your attending physician before starting this or any other new diet.* Once you've obtained clearance, be sure that you are monitored while on the diet, to ensure success.

Guidelines for the Modified Elimination Diet

1. Eliminate from your diet any foods that contain wheat, either in its whole or refined form, in breads, cereals, and pastas, or in the form of starch wheat-gluten, which is added to certain prepared foods. Also avoid foods that contain corn flour or corn meal. While it's a good idea to exclude all gluten-containing grains (e.g., spelt, kamut, oat, rye, barley, and malt), if this seems too restrictive, you can continue to eat them, but only in their whole forms. Foods made from rice, millet, buckwheat, potato, tapioca, arrowroot, or other gluten-free/corn-free flours are acceptable.

2. Eliminate all dairy foods (e.g., milk, cheese, yogurt, butter, and ice cream), as they contain the protein casein and lactose sugar. Avoid foods containing hydrogenated fats or trans fatty acids (e.g., margarine). Be careful of cheese and dairy substitutes (e.g., soy cheese), since they might contain casein and/or lactose. Those who find these restrictions too severe can eat organic dairy foods derived from goat or sheep milk once a week. Soy, rice, oat, almond (or other nut) beverages are acceptable.

3. Eliminate pork, beef, and veal. If this restriction is too much for you, you can have beef or veal once a week, but make sure that it is very lean. Avoid packaged, prepared, and/or procured meats (hot dogs, bologna, and most delicatessen meats). Chicken, turkey, lamb, and cold-water fresh fish are acceptable. Try to purchase meat from organically

raised (free of hormones and antibiotics, high-quality feed, free ranging) animals. Organic, free-range, omega-3–rich eggs are preferred (it is acceptable to have six per week). Naturally fermented, non-genetically modified soy protein is also fine; just don't consume it daily. With the exception of peanuts and pistachios, fresh, raw, salt-free (or very low salt) nuts and nut butters are acceptable. Always keep nuts and nut products in airtight containers in the fridge. Eat a variety of beans, as they are a good source of protein and fiber. Use unrefined, cold-pressed, natural plant oils rich in omega-3 and monounsaturated fatty acids (e.g., flaxseed, walnut, soy, olive, and Udo's Ultimate Oil Blend).

4. Completely avoid oranges, tomatoes, strawberries, and their juices, whether fresh-squeezed or otherwise, and avoid all dried fruits. It's also best to avoid eggplant, potatoes, and all types of bell peppers. If you wish to have vegetable or fruit juice from vegetables or fruits not mentioned above, make sure it's freshly squeezed, drink it immediately, and have no more than 12 ounces daily. Eat as much as you can of fresh raw vegetables and take two servings of fruit daily. Eat a variety of colorful vegetables and fruits, and wash them thoroughly of any pesticide residues.

5. Completely avoid alcohol, soda pop, and caffeine-containing beverages. However, if you must have coffee, choose an organic blend and have no more than 16 ounces a day, preferably without milk or sugar. Drink 6–8 glasses of pure water daily and as much high-quality, caffeine-free herbal tea as you like; if you find it hard to drink so much water, substitute some of the amount with the tea.

6. Eliminate foods that contain yeast and mold, monosodium glutamate (MSG), preservatives, food coloring, refined sugars, synthetic sweeteners, additives, synthetic agents, a lot of salt, trans fatty acids, and hydrogenated fats. In general, this means avoiding processed foods (packaged in cans, boxes, and plastic, etc.) and commercially prepared foods and condiments. Try making your own dressings and sauces. For instance, salad dressing can be made with olive oil, lemon, crushed garlic, fresh herbs, and spices. If you need to use sweeteners, you may sparingly use brown rice syrup, natural fruit sweeteners, fructose, and stevia. Brown sugar, raw cane sugar, honey, jams, molasses, maple syrup, corn syrup, and glucose-fructose syrup are all to be completely avoided.

APPENDIX 8.1
CORTISOL EVALUATION QUESTIONNAIRE

Medical

1. Do you have medically diagnosed depression that has lasted longer than six months?

Yes ☐ No ☐

2. Do you have difficulty falling asleep and/or do you wake up early?

Yes ☐ No ☐

3. Do you suffer from any chronic inflammatory condition (asthma, arthritis, migraines, etc.)?

Yes ☐ No ☐

4. Do you have an autoimmune disease (rheumatoid arthritis, lupus, Crohn's, etc.)?

Yes ☐ No ☐

5. Do you suffer from chronic year-round allergies?

Yes ☐ No ☐

6. Have you been diagnosed with hypothyroidism or any other thyroid disorder as an adult?

Yes ☐ No ☐

7. Do you have elevated cholesterol, blood pressure, and/or blood glucose?

Yes ☐ No ☐

Emotional

8. Do you feel anxious, overwhelmed, and easily frustrated about the responsibilities of your life on almost a daily basis?

Yes ☐ No ☐

9. Do you experience psychological or emotional conflict in dealing with your spouse, family members, friends, or co-workers on almost a daily basis?

Yes ☐ No ☐

10. Do you spend a significant portion of each day in constant worry and fear?

Yes ☐ No ☐

Physical

11. Do you suffer from frequent indigestion, poor elimination (less than one bowel movement a day), and/or peptic ulcer pain?

Yes ☐ No ☐

12. Have you steadily gained weight as you've aged, and/or are you unable to achieve permanent weight loss?

Yes ☐ No ☐

13. Are you constantly tired, and/or do you experience significant drops in energy as the day wears on?

Yes ☐ No ☐

14. Do you exercise less than 30 minutes per session three times a week?

Yes ☐ No ☐

15. Do you frequently get colds, flus, or cold sores, especially following periods of prolonged stress, and do you find it takes longer than usual to recover?

Yes ☐ No ☐

16. Do you have recurring or chronic infections?

Yes ☐ No ☐

17. Do you have a poorly healing wound?

Yes ☐ No ☐

18. Do you have adult acne or oily skin, especially on the upper body?

Yes ☐ No ☐

19. As you get older, do you find that you're developing an intolerance to more and more foods or that you're developing sensitivities to environmental agents like food additives (MSG), perfume, cleaning solvents, or other work-related chemicals?

Yes ☐ No ☐

20. Do you suffer from headaches at least once a week?

Yes ☐ No ☐

Social

21. Are you constantly rushing around, and/or are you always late for scheduled events?

Yes ☐ No ☐

22. Do you have difficulty saying no and often find yourself overcommitted?

Yes ☐ No ☐

Nutritional

23. Do you crave fatty, salty, and sweet junk food on almost a daily basis?

Yes ☐ No ☐

24. Do you have more than 2 ounces of alcohol or 20 ounces of caffeine-containing beverages a day?

Yes ☐ No ☐

25. Do you skip meals, give yourself less than 20 minutes to eat a meal, or eat at irregular times on a daily basis?

Yes ☐ No ☐

Interpretation

If you answered *yes* to

1 to 6 questions, you may have elevated cortisol levels.

7 to 12 questions, you have a very high probability of elevated cortisol.

13 to 25 questions, you are at very high risk of accelerated aging and associated diseases or of a progression of your current disease state.

APPENDIX 8.2
ADAPTOGENIC PHYTOMEDICINES AND THEIR FUNCTIONS

ADAPTOGENIC HERBS

American ginseng

Ashwagandha

Asian ginseng (panax ginseng)

Astragalus

Cordyceps

Holy basil

Jiaogulan

Maca

Reishi

Rhodiola

Schizandra

Siberian ginseng

Suma

Tribulus terrestris

FUNCTIONS

Protect against free-radical damage

Control excessive inflammation

Regulate blood sugar and cholesterol

Balance stress hormones

Strengthen nervous system and improve mood

Improve circulation

Protect liver and kidneys

Improve digestion and elimination

Increase energy and stamina

Improve sleep

Improve physical strength

Improve recovery

Promote a sense of well-being

Improve lung function

Improve immune function

Increase capacity for stress

Improve mental focus and concentration

APPENDIX 8.3
TAKING YOUR BASAL BODY TEMPERATURE

Purpose

Because thyroid hormones are required by every cell and tissue in the body to function properly, it's critical that your thyroid secrete the necessary hormones. Hypothyroidism, or low thyroid function, frequently goes undiagnosed by standard thyroid hormone blood tests. However, because well-regulated body temperature is directly controlled by your thyroid gland, a measurement of your basal body temperature gives a good indication of whether your thyroid gland is working optimally.

Procedure

Be sure to use a mercury thermometer, as digital thermometers are not as accurate. Before bed, shake down the thermometer to below 95°F (35°C).

As soon as you wake up in the morning, before getting out of bed, before eating or drinking anything, and before engaging in any activity, put the thermometer deep into your armpit. It's important that you make as little movement as possible. Leave the thermometer under your arm for 10 minutes, and then record the temperature. This measures your basal body temperature, generally the lowest temperature of the day.

Chart your temperature in this way every day for 90 days, at the same time each morning (between 6 a.m. and 8 a.m.).

Caution

Do not take your temperature when you have an infection, fever, or any other condition that might raise your temperature.

Women who are still menstruating should not take their temperature in the first three days of their cycle.

Interpretation

A normal basal body temperature is between 97.8°F and 98.2°F (36.5°C and 36.8°C). A basal body temperature of 97.2°F (36.2°C) or lower for 7 to 10 days is a strong indication of hypothyroidism. A 90-day average that is half a degree or more below the optimal range (i.e., an average of 97.5°F [36.9°C] or lower) may also indicate a high probability of hypothyroidism.

APPENDIX 9.1
QUESTIONNAIRE TO EVALUATE THE OVERGROWTH OF CANDIDA ALBICANS

Candida albicans is a yeast organism that commonly resides in the gastrointestinal tract. However, leaky gut syndrome, prolonged stress, weak immune function, medication use, food intolerances, poor dietary habits and lifestyle are among the major factors that can lead to over growth or a condition known as chronic candidiasis. When overgrowth occurs, this yeast and its toxic by-products can cause gastrointestinal disorders as well as allergies, chronic inflammatory disorders and fatigue. The endocrine, immune and nervous systems are also usually affected when this fungus becomes a systemic problem.

Following is a questionnaire that will help you determine whether chronic candidiasis may be an existing problem for you.

If the candida still exists after following recommendations in Chapter 9, consider consulting a healthcare practitioner experienced in treating chronic candidiasis.

Questionnaire

History

1. Have you taken antibiotics for acne or any other condition for one month or longer?

Yes ☐ No ☐

2. Have you taken more than 10 rounds of antibiotics up to this point in your life? (A round means an antibiotic was taken for the duration of one week. Thus, 10-day therapy counts for one and a half rounds and two-week therapy counts for two rounds, and so on.)

Yes ☐ No ☐

3. Have you taken birth control pills or other hormone-based medications for more than two years on a continuous basis?

Yes ☐ No ☐

4. Have you taken prednisone or other steroid-based medications for more than one month on a continuous basis?

Yes ☐ No ☐

5. Have you taken non-steroidal medications for more than six months on a continuous basis?

Yes ☐ No ☐

6. Have you taken antacids, H2 blockers, or proton pump inhibitors (medications that block stomach acids) for more than six months on a continuous basis?

Yes ☐ No ☐

7. Do you seem to be bothered by or react strongly to any one of following environmental agents: chemicals, detergents, dust, grasses, molds, mildew, perfumes, pesticides, pollution, pollen, ragweed, trees, or tobacco smoke?

Yes ☐ No ☐

8. Do you have allergies, intolerances, or sensitivities to foods (e.g., milk, wheat, peanuts) and food additives (e.g., MSG, coloring agents, preservatives) that manifest either in the gastrointestinal tract or systemically?

Yes ☐ No ☐

9. Do you have unresolved or problematic athlete's foot, ringworm, jock itch, psoriasis, or other infections of the skin or nails?

Yes ☐ No ☐

10. Do you have chronic or recurring infections such as cystitis (bladder), prostatitis, sinusitis, or vaginal yeast infections?

Yes ☐ No ☐

11. Do you crave sugar, sweet foods, or desserts?

Yes ☐ No ☐

12. Do you crave breads?

Yes ☐ No ☐

13. Do you crave alcohol?

Yes ☐ No ☐

Digestive Tract

14. Do you experience constipation or diarrhea?

Yes ☐ No ☐

15. Do you have excessive gas, bloating, or abdominal distension?

Yes ☐ No ☐

16. Do you have frequent heartburn or indigestion after meals?

Yes ☐ No ☐

17. Do you have irritable bowel syndrome?

Yes ☐ No ☐

18. Do you have very foul-smelling stools and or mucus in the stools?

Yes ☐ No ☐

19. Do you have hemorrhoids?

Yes ☐ No ☐

20. Do you have chronic or recurring canker sores or mouth blisters?

Yes ☐ No ☐

21. Do you have foul breath and/or a coated tongue?

Yes ☐ No ☐

Upper and Lower Respiratory Tract and Related Mucous Membranes

22. Do you have chronic postnasal drip, nasal congestion (especially in the morning upon awakening) and/or dry nasal passages and/or feel itchy?

Yes ☐ No ☐

23. Do you have a chronic productive cough (producing phlegm) and/or wheezing, shortness of breath, and tightness in the chest?

Yes ☐ No ☐

24. Do you have chronic urinary urgency, frequency, and/or burning and/or cloudy urine?

Yes ☐ No ☐

25. Do you have chronic burning, tearing, or dry eyes and/or blurry vision?

Yes ☐ No ☐

26. Do you have ear pressure, pain, and/or chronic fluid buildup in your ears?

Yes ☐ No ☐

Muscles, Joints, Skin, and Other Related Connective Tissue

27. Do you have chronic muscular aches and/or weakness?

Yes ☐ No ☐

28. Do you have joint pain or swelling, especially in the morning upon awakening?

Yes ☐ No ☐

29. Do you have itchy skin (also in vaginal and rectal areas), skin rashes, eczema, or psoriasis?

Yes ☐ No ☐

30. Do you have acne, especially on the upper body?

Yes ☐ No ☐

Central Nervous System

31. Do you have frequent mood swings, irritability, or depression?

Yes ☐ No ☐

32. Do you have poor memory, focus, feel hazy, hungover, spacy and/or become easily mentally fatigued?

Yes ☐ No ☐

33. Do you have numbness, tingling, or burning in the extremities?

Yes ☐ No ☐

34. Do you have chronic headaches, pressure, or a congested feeling?

Yes ☐ No ☐

35. Do you experience dizziness, loss of balance, or incoordination?

Yes ☐ No ☐

Metabolism and Hormones

36. Do you always feel fatigued and physically drained despite getting an adequate amount of sleep?

Yes ☐ No ☐

37. Do you have hypoglycemia reactions (nervousness, jitteriness, light-headedness, etc.) despite eating on a regular basis?

Yes ☐ No ☐

38. Do you often feel drowsy or sleep during the day, especially after eating?

Yes ☐ No ☐

39. Do you accumulate fluid in your tissues and feel puffy or heavy as the day wears on?

Yes ☐ No ☐

40. Do you have cumbersome or painful menstrual periods?

Yes ☐ No ☐

41. Do you have cysts in the breast or ovaries or do you have endometriosis?

Yes ☐ No ☐

Immune System

42. Do you have poor resistance to infection, recover slowly, and/or have swollen lymph nodes and glands?

Yes ☐ No ☐

Interpretation

If you answered *yes* to 2 or more of the first 13 questions and to 14 or more of the next 29 questions, there is a strong possibility that you have chronic candidiasis for which you need treatment.

APPENDIX 9.2 APPLYING THE 4R PROGRAM IN OPTIMIZING GASTROINTESTINAL FUNCTION AND OVERALL HEALTH

The 4R Gastrointestinal Restoration Program was developed by the research team at Metagenics and taught by the Institute for Functional Medicine to health-care practitioners at their clinical courses. (See Appendix 7.1.) This program was designed for individuals with functional gastrointestinal disorders, chronic inflammatory disorders, and who are chronically unwell with problematic health. Although the 4R program requires a great deal of effort and patience, as it has you going beyond the steps outlined in Chapter 9, it offers innumerable rewards.

The 4R Program

Step 1: The First "R" – Remove

This first step involves removing pathogenic bacteria, fungi, viruses, parasites, other environmentally derived toxins, gut-derived toxins, and food sensitivities from your intestinal tract and your system. The essence of this first step is to enhance the detoxification process carried out by your liver, intestines, and kidneys in order to remove toxins, by eliminating the foods that may cause the most strain on your system. Strict adherence to the Elimination Diet mentioned in Chapter 7 and outlined in Appendix 7.2 is critical.

Start Step 1 by taking UltraClear or UltraClear PLUS (ideal for those with multiple chemical sensitivities) or UltraInflamX – UltraInflavogen in Canada – (ideal for those with chronic inflammatory disorders), which are all distributed by Metagenics. (See Appendix 7.1.)

> ½ scoop of one of these products mixed in water or rice milk twice daily on an empty stomach before or in between meals for 3 days.
> 1 scoop twice daily for 7 days.
> 2 scoops twice daily for 7–14 days.
> 2 scoops three times daily for 7–14 days.
> 2 scoops five times daily for 3–5 days (those who can afford to lose weight and are able to go without solid food need only rely on the drink at this stage for the 3–5 days period).
> 2 scoops three times daily for 7–14 days.
> 2 scoops twice daily for 7–14 days.

Be sure to drink 6–8 glasses of pure water and take supplemental fiber morning and night while on this regime to ensure full elimination of toxins. The phytomedicinal cleansing formulas mentioned in Chapter 9 can be added if you need additional support. Those with confirmed pathogenic bacteria, fungi, or parasites should add a broad-spectrum anti-microbial phytomedicinal formula while doing this step.

Step 2: The Second "R" – Replace

Step 2 will bring your digestive enzymes back to the higher levels needed to ensure proper breakdown and assimilation of food. Select a high-quality digestive enzyme supplement, as mentioned in Chapter 9. Those who have difficulty digesting protein-rich foods should select an enzyme that has hydrochloric acid as additional support.

If digestion doesn't improve, even after increasing the dosage, or if they stop working after a while, take liquid herbal bitters instead, as mentioned in Chapter 9. Taking herbal bitters will stimulate digestive secretions as well as increase the production of saliva in the mouth, thereby preventing bacterial overgrowth that causes dry mouth, foul breath, gum disease, and tooth decay.

Step 2 should take at least one month before results are noticed. Keep in mind that by supporting the digestive process, you are helping your system to absorb more of the nutrients contained in high-quality food. Also, thoroughly pulverized food is less likely to cause leaky gut syndrome. Furthermore, enzymatic support controls the growth of pathogenic micro-organisms.

Step 3: The Third "R" – Reinoculate

In this step, you reintroduce into your body beneficial bacteria (probiotics) and factors that promote their growth (prebiotics). (The merits of probiotics have been discussed in Chapter 9.) Fructo-oligosaccharides (FOS) are an example of prebiotics: they are a special type of sugar that is a food source of beneficial bacteria. Remember to take your probiotics at the beginning of all meals. Step 3 has to be followed for at least two months before benefits can be expected. Consider taking supplemental probiotics on a permanent basis, to help you meet the numerous challenges that throw off gut flora. When picking your probiotic, remember that some probiotics work specifically in the large intestine to promote regularity, others work in the small intestine to improve digestion, and others work in both areas, so find the formula that suits your needs.

Step 4: The Fourth "R" – Regenerate

In this step, you assist the regeneration of gut mucosa (the lining of the stomach and of the small and large intestines). This is done by adding factors that help support the intestinal immune system, control intestinal inflammation, and ultimately ensure the repair of damaged epithelial tissue (the cells that line the digestive tract). This fourth step is essential if you hope to establish the resilient kind of health needed in today's world of excessive stress and toxicity. It's especially important for those with leaky gut syndrome.

Take UltraClear Sustain® (called UltraClear GI in Canada) like the products in Step 1. UltraClear Sustain differs from the other powders in that it is rich in the amino acid L-glutamine, which is needed for the nourishment of the cells of the gut.

Take an essential fatty acid (EFA) supplement that combines an ideal ratio of omega-6 and omega-3 fatty acids, such as 2 tablespoonsful or more of Udo's Ultimate Oil Blend® daily with meals. Taking EFAs helps to control intestinal inflammation, strengthens the intestinal immune system, and ultimately helps to regenerate a healthy gut.

Take a mixed tocopherol form of natural-sourced vitamin E. Take one 400 IU capsule twice daily with meals to stimulate immune function, control inflammation, and protect the gut from free-radical damage.

Mix 2 tablespoons of Endefen™ powder, (distributed by Metagenics; see Appendix 7.1), in water twice daily. This product contains several natural ingredients that complement the above recommendations and also ensure successful regeneration of the gut.

Additional Comments

The 4R program can be done one step at a time in order to be able to evaluate the benefit of each step before moving on to the next one. After completing Step 1, however Steps 2 and 3 or 2, 3, and 4 may be combined and done at once. Continuing with supplemental fiber is always a good idea for Steps 2, 3, and 4, although it may be reduced in Step 4, since Endefen™ contains fiber. The time taken for each step whether combined or not varies on an individual basis. It is also important to continue to follow the Modified Elimination Diet during all four steps.

Conclusion

As you can see, the 4R Program is quite ambitious, and it will take at least four months to complete it. However, ultimately you will create a strong foundation of health. The gut is, literally, ground zero. Good health can only be built on a healthy gut.

REFERENCE NOTES

Introduction

1. Fries, J.F. Aging, natural death, and the compression of morbidity. *N Engl J Med* 303.3 (1980): 130–35; Vita, A.J., et al. Aging, health risks and cumulative disability. *N Engl J Med* 338.15 (1998): 1035–41.

Chapter 1 Perspectives on Health and Aging

1. U.S. Department of Health and Human Services. Table 12: Estimated life expectancy at birth in years, by race and sex: Death Registration States, 1900–1928 and United States, 1929–1997. *National Vital Statistics Report* 47.28. Hyattsville, MD, 1999.

2. Statistics Canada. *Compendium of Vital Statistics 1996,* Cat. No. 84-214-XPE. Ottawa, 1999.

3. Heart and Stroke Foundation of Canada. *Heart Disease and Stroke in Canada.* Ottawa, 1997; U.S. Department of Health and Human Services. National Vital Statistics Report. *Deaths: Leading Causes for 1999.* Hyattsville, MD, 2001. 49(11).

4. National Cancer Institute of Canada. *Canadian Cancer Statistics 1998.* Toronto, 1998.

5. Health Canada, Diabetes Division. *Diabetes in Canada: National Statistics and Opportunities for Improved Surveillance, Prevention and Control.* Ottawa, 1999.

6. Statistics Canada. *National Population Health Survey, 1996–1997.* Special tabulations. Ottawa, 1998.

Chapter 2 Why and How We Age

1. Timbrel, J.A. *Principles of Biochemical Toxicology.* 2nd ed. Washington, DC: Taylor and Francis, 1992.

2. Hayflick, L. *How and Why We Age.* New York: Ballantine Books, a division of Random House, 1994. 236.

3. Glutathione and morbidity in a community-based sample of elderly. *Clin Epidemiol* 47.9 (1994 Sept): 1021–26.

4. Bradlow, H.L., et al. Phytochemicals as modulators of cancer risk. *Adv Exp Med Biol* 472 (1999): 207–21; Joshipura, K.J., F.B. Hu, and J.E. Manson. The effect of fruit and vegetable intake on risk for coronary heart disease. *Ann Intern Med* 134.12 (2001): 1106–14; Gann, P.H., et al. Lower prostate cancer risk in men with elevated plasma lycopene levels: results of a prospective analysis. *Cancer Res* 59.6 (15 March 1999): 1225–30; Longnecker, M.P., et al. Intake of carrots, spinach, and supplements containing vitamin A in relation to risk of breast cancer. *Epidemiol Biomarkers Prev* 6.11 (Nov. 1997): 887–97; Steinmetz, K.A., et al. Vegetables, fruit, and cancer prevention: a review. *J Am Diet Assoc* 96.10 (Oct. 1996): 1027–39; Snodderly, D.M. Evidence for protection against age-related macular degeneration by carotenoids and antioxidant vitamins. *Am J Clin Nutr* 62.6 suppl. (Dec. 1995): 1448S–61S.

5. Stephens, N.G., et al. Randomized controlled trial of vitamin E in patients with coronary disease: Cambridge Heart Antioxidant Study (CHAOS). *Lancet* 347 (1996): 781–86; Langsjoen, P.H., S.

Vadhanavikit, and K. Folkers. Effective treatment with coenzyme Q10 of patients with chronic myocardial disease. *Drugs Exptl Clin Res* 11 (1985): 577–79; LeBars, P.L., et al. A placebo-controlled, double-blind, randomized trial of an extract of ginkgo biloba for dementia. *JAMA* 278.16 (1997): 1327–32; Packer, L. The role of anti-oxidative treatment of diabetes mellitus. *Diabetologia* 36 (1993): 1212–13; Cholesterol-lowering effect of soy protein. *Am J Clin Nutr* 68.6, suppl. S (1998): 1380S–84S; Lamartiniere, C.A., J.X. Zhang, and M.S. Cotroneo. Gerstein studies in rats: potential for breast cancer prevention and reproductive and developmental toxicity. *Am J Clin Nutr* 68.6, suppl. S (1998): 1400S–1405S; Soy protein lipids and bone density in postmenopausal women. *Am J Clin Nutr* 68.6, suppl. S (1998): 1375S–79S; Combs, G.F., Jr. et al. Reduction of cancer mortality and incidence by selenium supplementation. *Med Klin* 92.3, suppl. (15 Sept. 1997): 42–45; Klipstein-Grobusch, Kerstin, et al. Dietary antioxidants and risk of myocardial infarction in the elderly: the Rotterdam Study. *Am J Clin Nutr* 69.2 (Feb. 1999): 261–66; Schmidt, R., et al. Plasma antioxidants and cognitive performance in middle-aged and older adults: results of the Austrian Stroke Prevention Study. *J Am Geriatr Soc* 46.11 (Nov. 1998): 1407–10; De la Fuente, M., et al. Immune function in aged women is improved by ingestion of vitamins C and E. *Can J Physiol Pharmacol* 76.4 (April 1998): 373–80; Galley, H.F., et al. Combination oral antioxidant supplementation reduced blood pressure. *Clin Sci (Colch)* 92.4 (April 1997): 361–65; Wilkinson, I.B., et al. Oral vitamin C reduces arterial stiffness and platelet aggregation in humans. *J Cardiovasc Pharmacol* 34.5 (Nov. 1999): 690–93.

6. Luft, R. The development of mitochondrial medicine. *Proct Natl Acad Sci USA* 91 (1994): 8731–38; Wallace, D.C. Mitochondrial genetics: a paradigm for aging and degenerative diseases. *Science* 256 (1992): 628–32.

7. McCarty, M.F. An expanded concept of "insurance" supplementation—broad-spectrum protection from cardiovascular disease. *Med Hypotheses* 7 (1981): 11287–302; Carta, A., et al. Acetyl-L-carnitine and Alzheimer's disease: pharmacological considerations beyond the cholinergic sphere. *Ann N Y Acad Sci* 695 (1993): 324–26; Barbiroli, B., et al. Lipoic (thiotic) acid increases brain energy availability and skeletal muscle performance as shown by in vivo 31 p-mrs in a patient with mitochondrial cytopathy. *J Neurol* 242 (1995): 472–77; Crane, F.L., I.L. Sun, and E.E. Sun. The essential functions of coenzyme Q. *Clin Investig* 71 (1993): S55–59; Miquel, J., et al. N-acetylcysteine protects against age-related decline of oxidative phosphorylation in liver mitochondria. *Eur J Pharmacol* 292 (1995): 333–35.

8. Pizzorno, J.E., and M.T. Murray. "Immune Support." In *Encyclopedia of Natural Medicine*. Rocklin, CA: Prima Publishing, 1991; Hadden, J.W., et al. Thymic involution in aging; prospects for correction. *Ann NY Acyad Sci* 673 (1992): 231–39.

Chapter 3 Saboteurs of Health

1. McGinnis, J.M., and W.H. Foege. Actual causes of death in the United States. *JAMA* 270 (1993): 2207–12.

2. Centers for Disease Control and Prevention. Cigarette smoking-attributable mortality and years of potential life lost—United States, 1984. *Morbidity and Mortality Weekly Report* 46 (1997): 444–50.

3. Peto, R., et al. *Mortality from Smoking in Developed Countries 1950–2000*. New York: Oxford University Press, 1994.

4. U.S. Department of Health and Human Services. *Reducing the Health Consequences of Smoking: 25 Years of Progress*. A Report of the Surgeon General. Atlanta, GA: U.S. Department of Health and Human Services, Public Health Service, Centers for Disease Control and Prevention, Center for Chronic Disease Prevention and Health Promotion, Office on Smoking and Health, 1989.

5. Centers for Disease Control and Prevention. Youth risk behavior surveillance—United States, 1999. *Morbidity and Mortality Weekly Report* 49 (2000).

6. National Library of Medicine, National Institute of Health. 27 July 2001 <www.nlm.nih.gov/medlineplus/ency/article/002393.htm>.

7. Selye, H. *The Stress of Life.* 2nd ed. McGraw-Hill, 1978.

8. "How Does Stress Affect Us?" Help Center, American Psychological Association. 28 Sept. 2001 <helping.apa.org/work/stress2.html>.

9. Cohen, S., D.A. Tyrrell, and A.P. Smith. Negative life events, perceived stress, negative affect, and susceptibility to the common cold. *J Pers Soc Psychol* 64.1 (1993): 131–40.

10. Van Cauter, E., R. Leproult, L. Plat. Age-related changes in slow wave sleep and REM sleep and relationship with growth hormone and cortisol levels in healthy men. *JAMA* 284.7 (2000): 861–68.

11. "The Importance of Sleep." National Sleep Foundation. 18 Sept. 2001 <www.sleepfoundation.org/about/html>.

12. Weindruch, R., and R. Walford. *The Retardation of Aging and Disease by Dietary Restriction.* Springfield, IL: Charles C. Thomas, 1988.

13. National Institute of Health. National Institute of Aging: In Search of the Secrets of Aging. 27 July 2001 <www.nia.nih.gov/health/pubs/secrets percent2Dof percent2Daging/p4.htm#p41>.

14. McGinnis, J., and W. Foege. Actual causes of death in the United States. *JAMA* 270.18 (1993): 2208.

15. Alcohol Epidemiologic Data System. *Surveillance Report #54: Liver Cirrhosis Mortality in the United States, 1970–97,* by F. Saadatmand et al. Rockville, MD: National Institute on Alcohol Abuse and Alcoholism, Division of Biometry and Epidemiology, Dec. 2000; National Institute on Alcohol Abuse and Alcoholism, *Alcohol Research & Health* 17.2 (1993): 133–76; National Institute on Alcohol Abuse and Alcoholism, *Alcohol Alert,* no. 21 (July 1993); National Institute on Alcohol Abuse and Alcoholism, *Alcohol Alert,* no. 26 (Nov. 1995).

16. Kubota, M., et al. Alcohol and brain aging. *Journal of Neurology, Neurosurgery and Psychiatry* 71 (2001): 104–6.

17. U.S. Department of Agriculture and U.S. Department of Health and Human Services. *Nutrition and Your Health: Dietary Guidelines for Americans.* Rockville, MD, 1995. 40.

18. Gaziano, J.M., et al. Moderate alcohol intake, increased levels of high-density lipoprotein and its subfractions, and decreased risk of myocardial infarction. *N Engl J Med* 329 (1993): 1829–34.

19. Gordon, T., et al. Alcohol and high-density lipoprotein cholesterol. *Circulation* 64, suppl III (1981): 63–67.

Chapter 4 Measurements of Successful Aging

1. Perls, T.T., M.H. Silver, and J.F. Lauerman. *Living to 100 (Lessons in Living to Your Maximum Potential at Any Age).* New York: Basic Books, 1999.

2. Ibid.

3. Allard, M., V. Lebre, and J.M. Robine. *The Longest Life: The 122 Extraordinary Years of Jeanne Calment, from Van Gogh's Time to Ours.* New York: W.H. Freeman, 1998; Erikson, E., J.M. Erikson, and H.Q. Kivnick. *Vital Involvement in Old Age: The Experience of Old Age in Our Time.* New York: W.W. Norton, 1986; Higgins, G.O. *Resilient Adults: Overcoming a Cruel Past.* San Francisco: Jossey-

Bass, 1994; Lowenthal, M.F., and C. Haven. "Interaction and Adaptation: Intimacy as a Critical Variable." In *Middle Age and Aging*, edited by B.L. Neugarten. Chicago: University of Chicago Press, 1968. 390–400; Fry, W.E. "Humor, Physiology and the Aging Process." In *Humor and Aging*, edited by L. Nehamow, K.A. McCluskey-Fawcett, and P.E. McGhee. New York: Academic Press, 1986. 81–98; Benson, H., with M. Stark. *Timeless Healing: The Power and Biology of Belief*. New York: Simon & Schuster, 1997; Koenig, H.G. Research on religion and mental health in later life: a review and commentary. *J Geriatr Psychiatry* 23 (1990): 23–53; Berkman, L.F. The role of social relations in health promotion. *Psychosom Med* 57 (1995): 245–54.

4. Sapolsky, R.M. *Why Zebras Don't Get Ulcers: An Updated Guide to Stress, Stress-Reduced Diseases, and Coping*. New York: W.H. Freeman, 1998.

5. Agarwal, S., and R.S. Sohal. Relationship between susceptibility to protein oxidation, aging, and maximum life span potential of different species. *Exp Gerentol* 31 (1996): 365–72; Martin, G.M., S.N. Austad, and T.E. Johnson. Genetic analysis of aging: role of oxidative damage and environmental stresses. *Nat Genet* 13 (1996): 25; Kapur, N. *Managing Your Memory: A Self-Help Memory Manual for Improving Everyday Memory Skills*. Gaylord, MI: National Rehabilitation Services, 1991; Lapp, D.C. *Don't Forget! Easy Exercises for a Better Memory at Any Age*. New York: McGraw-Hill Paperbacks, 1996.

6. Perls, *Living to 100*.

Chapter 5 Creating Emotional Balance

1. Statistics Canada. *Health Reports, How Healthy Are Canadians? 2001 Annual Report*. Cat. No. 82-003-XIE. Ottawa: Canadian Institute for Health Education, 2001. 21–31.

2. Duxbury, L., and C. Higgins. "Work Network—Work-Life Balance in the New Millennium: Where Are We? Where Do We Need to Go?" Canadian Policy Research Networks Discussion Paper No. W/12 (2001): 14.

3. National Institute of Mental Health. "Mental Illness in America: The Numbers Count" <www.nimh.nih.gov>. Science on Our Minds Fact Sheet Series. 10 March 2002 <www.nimh.nih.gov/publicat/numbers.cfm>.

4. Canadian Psychological Association. "Psychological Treatment Works for Depression" <www.cpa.ca>. Psychological Treatment Works Fact Sheet. 10 March 2002 <www.cpa.ca/factsheets/depression.htm>.

5. American Psychological Association. "How Does Stress Affect Us?" <www.apa.org>. APA Online, adapted from *The Stress Solution* by Lyle H. Miller and Alma Dell Smith. 10 March 2002 <www.helping.apa.org/work/stress2.html>.

6. Johns Hopkins Medical Institutions. "Positive Attitude Is Best Prevention against Heart Disease" <www.hopkinsmedicine.org>. Press release. 15 February 2002 <www.hopkinsmedicine.org/press/2001/NOVEMBER/011112.htm>.

7. Snowdon, D. *Aging with Grace, What the Nun Study Teaches Us about Leading Longer, Healthier and More Meaningful Lives*. New York: Bantam Books, 2001.

8. Parrott, A. Does cigarette smoking cause stress? *Am Psychol* 54 (1999): 817–20.

9. Mayo Foundation for Medical Education and Research, "Spirituality and Chronic Pain." 15 February 2002 <www.mayoclinic.com>. MayoClinic.com <www.mayoclinic.com/findinformation/conditioncenters/invoke.cfm?objectid=67A79059-32B9-4A7D-AA413F254B235FD1>.

10. Benson, H. *Timeless Healing: The Power and Biology of Belief.* New York: Scribner, 1996.

11. Pargament, K.I., et al. Religious struggle as a predicator of mortality among medically ill elderly patients. *Arch Int Med* 161 (2001): 1881–85.

Chapter 6 Exercising Your Way to a Younger Body

1. Kwasnicki, S. *Go for Fit: The Winning Way to Fat Loss.* Vancouver, BC: Raincoast Books, 1999. 62.

2. Penninx, B.W., et al. Physical exercise and the prevention of disability in activities of daily living in older persons with osteoarthritis. *Arch Int Med* 161 (2001): 2309–16.

3. Flatarone, M. U.S. Department of Agriculture. Human Nutrition Center on Aging. Tufts University. Paper presented at House Select Committee on Aging, Feb. 1991.

4. Health Canada. *Canada's Physical Activity Guide to Healthy Active Living for Older Adults.* Cat. No. H39-429/1999-2E. Ottawa. 4.

5. Drink more water. *IDEA Personal Trainer* May 2000: 60.

6. Kwasnicki. *Go for Fit.* 98.

7. Ibid.

8. Strength training when you are 50+. *IDEA Health and Fitness Source* May 2000: 88.

Chapter 7 Nutrition for Optimal Health

1. Anderson, J.W., B.M. Johnstone, and M.E. Cook-Newell. Meta-analysis of the effects of soy protein intake on serum lipids. *N Engl J Med* 333 (1995): 276–82; Potter, S.M., et al. Soy protein and isoflavones: their effects on blood lipids and bone density in postmenopausal women. *Am J Clin Nutr* 68, suppl. (1991): 1375S–79S.

2. Krauss, R.M., et al. AHA Scientific Statement, AHA Dietary Guidelines, Revision 2000: A Statement for Healthcare Professionals from the Nutrition Committee of the American Heart Association. *Circulation* 102 (2000): 2284.

3. National Research Council, Food and Nutrition Board. *Recommended Dietary Allowances.* 10th ed. Washington, DC: National Academy Press, 1989.

4. Goff, J., S. Gropper, and S. Hunt. *Advanced Nutrition and Human Metabolism.* New York: West Publishing Co., 1995.

5. Dreon, D.M., et al. Low-density lipoprotein subclass patterns and lipoprotein response to a reduced-fat diet in men. *FASEB Journal* 8 (1994): 121–26; Starc, T.J., et al. Greater dietary intake of simple carbohydrate is associated with lower concentrations of high-density lipoprotein cholesterol in hypercholesterolemic children. *Am J Clin Nutr* 67 (1998): 1147–54.

6. Rimm, E.B., et al. Vegetable, fruit, and cereal fibre intake and risk of coronary heart disease among men. *JAMA* 275 (1996): 447–51; Jacobs, D.R., Jr., et al. Whole grain intake may reduce the risk of ischemic heart disease death in postmenopausal women: the Iowa Women's Health Study. *Am J Clin Nutr* 68 (1998): 248–57.; Anderson J.W., B.M. Smith, and N.J. Gustafson. Health benefits and practical aspects of high-fibre diets. *Am J Clin Nutr* 59 (1994): 1242S–47S.

7. American Heart Association, "Carbohydrates and Sugars," 10 June 2002 <216.185.112.5/presenter.jhtml?identifier=4471>.

8. Albert, C.M., et al. Fish consumption and risk of sudden cardiac death. *JAMA* 279 (1998): 23–28; Siscovick, D.S., et al. Dietary intake and cell membrane levels of long-chain n-3 polyunsaturated fatty acids and the risk of primary cardiac arrest. *JAMA* 274 (1995): 1363–67; Harris, W.S. N-3 fatty acids and serum lipoproteins: human studies. *Am J Clin Nutr* 65 (1997): 1645S–54S; Mori, T.A., et al. Interactions between dietary fat, fish, and fish oils and their effects on platelet function in men at risk of cardiovascular disease. *Arterioscler Thomb Vasc Biol* 17 (1997): 279–86; Guallar, E., et al. Omega-3 fatty acids in adipose tissue and risk of myocardial infarction: the EURAMIC Study. *Arterioscler Thromb Vasc Biol* 19 (1999): 1111–18.

9. Krauss et al. AHA Scientific Statement. 2284.

10. Keys, A., J.T. Anderson, and F. Grande. Serum cholesterol response to changes in diet, IV, particular saturated fatty acids in the diet. *Metabolism* 14 (1965): 776–87; Hegsted, D.M., et al. Quantitative effects of dietary fat on serum cholesterol in man. *Am J Clin Nutr* 17 (1965): 281–95. Golay, A., and E. Bobbioni. The role of dietary fat in obesity. *Int J Obes* 21.S3 (1997): S2–S11; Bruce, W.R., T.M. Wolever, and A. Giacca. Mechanisms linking diet and colorectal cancer: the possible role of insulin resistance. *Nutr Cancer* 37.1 (2000): 19–26.

11. Lichtenstein, A.H. Trans fatty acids, plasma lipid levels, and risk of developing cardiovascular disease. *Circulation* 95 (1997): 2588–90.

12. Judd, J.T., et al. Dietary trans fatty acids: effects on plasma lipids and lipoproteins of healthy men and women [see comments]. *Am J Clin Nutr* 59 (1994): 861–68; Lichtenstein, A.H., et al. Effects of different forms of dietary hydrogenated fats on serum lipoprotein cholesterol levels [see comments; published erratum appears in *N Engl J Med* 341 (1999): 856]. *N Engl J Med* 340 (1999): 1933–40.

13. Kohlmeier, L. et al. Adipose tissue trans fatty acids and breast cancer in the European Community multicenter study on antioxidants, myocardial infarction, and breast cancer. *Cancer Epidemiol Biomarkers Prev* 6.9 (1997): 705–10; Holmes, M.D. Association of dietary intake of fat and fatty acids with risk of breast cancer. *J Amer Med Assoc* 281.10 (1999): 914–20.

14. Shekelle, R.B., and J. Stamler. Dietary cholesterol and ischaemic heart disease [see comments]. *Lancet* 1 (1989): 1177–79.

15. American Heart Association, "A Statement for Healthcare Professionals from the AHA Task Force on Risk Reduction." 13 June 2002 <216.185.112.5/presenter.jhtml?identifier=1807>.

16. "Background on Functional Foods." International Food Information Council Foundation. Washington, DC. 29 Oct. 2002 <ific.org/proactive/newsroom/release.vtml?id=18801>.

17. Agency for Healthcare Research and Quality (AHRQ) Evidence Report/Technology Assessment, No. 20. 23 Feb. 2002 <www.ahrq.gov/clinic/garlicsum.htm>.

18. Verdery, R.B., et al. Calorie restriction increases HDL2 levels in rhesus monkeys. *Am J Physiol* 273 (1997): E714–19.

19. Lane, M.A., et al. Dehydroepiandrosterone sulfate: a biomarker of primate aging slowed by calorie restriction. *J Clin Endocrinol Metab* 82 (1997): 2093–96.

20. Burke, G.L., et al. Factors associated with healthy aging: the Cardiovascular Health Study. *J Am Geriatr Soc* 49 (2001): 254–62.

21. Fact Sheet: Food Allergy and Intolerances. National Institute of Allergy and Infectious Diseases, National Institute of Health, Bethesda, MD, 25 June 2001. 12 March 2002 <www.niaid.nih.gov/factsheets/food.htm>.

Chapter 8 The Role of Hormones

1. Murray, M.T. *The Healing Power of Herbs.* Rocklin, CA: Prima Publishing, 1992. 277–78; Brekhman II and Dardymov IV. New substances of plant origin which increase nonspecific resistance. *Annu Rev Pharmacol* 9 (1969): 419–30; Petkov, W. Pharmacological studies of the drug P Ginseng C.A. Meyer. *Arzniemittel-Forsch* 9 (1959): 305–11; D'Angelo, L., et al. A double-blind, placebo controlled clinical study on the effect of a standardized ginseng extract on psychomotor performance in healthy volunteers. *J Ethnopharmacol* 16 (1986): 15–22; Bombardelli, E., A. Cirstoni, and A. Lietti. "The effect of acute and chronic (Panax) ginseng saponins treatment on adrenal function; biochemical and pharmacological." Proceedings of the 3rd International Ginseng Symposium, Korean Ginseng Research Institute, 1980. 9–16; Fulder, S.J. Ginseng and the hypothalamic-pituitary control of stress. *Am J Chin Med* 9 (1981): 112–18.

2. Mowrey, D.B. *Herbal Tonic Therapies.* New Canaan, CN: Keats Publishing, 1993.

3. Institute of Medicine. *Dietary Reference Intakes for Vitamin C, Vitamin E, Selenium and Carotenoids. Institute of Medicine.* Washington DC: National Academy Press, 2000; Institute of Medicine. *Dietary Reference Intakes for Thiamin, Riboflavin, Niacin, Vitamin B6, Folate, Vitamin B12, Pantothenic Acid, Biotin and Choline.* Washington DC: National Academy Press, 1998.

4. Ibid.

5. Ringsdorf, W.M., Jr., and E. Cheraskin. Optimal nutrition: a new prescription. *J Pedod* 8.2 (Winter 1984): 123–37.

Chapter 9 Digestion: The Fast Track to Good Health

1. Kelly, G.S. Hydrochloric acid: physiological functions and clinical implications. *Altern Med Rev* 2 (1997): 116–27.

2. Catanzaro, J.A., and L. Green. Microbial ecology and dysbiosis in human medicine. *Altern Med Rev* 2 (1997): 202–9, 196–305.

3. Liska, D.J., D. Lukaczer. Gut dysfunction and chronic disease: the benefits of applying the 4R GI Restoration Program. *Applied Nutritional Science Reports.* MET558. San Clemente, CA, 2001.

4. Ibid.

5. Gaby, A.R. The role of hidden food allergy/intolerance in chronic disease. *Altern Med Rev* 3 (1998): 90–100.

6. Sherman, J.A. *The Complete Botanical Prescriber.* 3rd ed. Self-published. 1993.

7. Johnson, B., and R. McIssac. Effect of some anti-ulcer agents on mucosal blood flow. *Br J Pharmacol* 1 (308): 1981; Kassir, Z.A. Endoscopic controlled trial of four drug regimens in the treatment of chronic duodenal ulceration. *Irish Med J* 78 (1985): 153–56; Turpie, A.G., J. Runcie, and T.J. Thomson. Clinical trial of deglycyrrhizinated liquorice in gastric ulcer. *Gut* 10 (1969): 299–303.

8. Huwez, F.U., et al. Mastic gum kills helicobacter pylori. *N Engl J Med* 339 (1998): 1946; Huwez, F.U., and M.J. Al-Habbal. Mastic in treatment of benign gastric ulcers. *Gastroenterol Japon* 21 (1986): 273–74; Al-Habbal, M.J., Z. Al-Habbal, and F.U. Huwez. A double-blind controlled clinical trial of mastic and placebo in the treatment of duodenal ulcer. *J Clin Exp Pharm Physiol* 11 (1984): 541–44.

9. Al-Said, M.S., et al. Evaluation of mastic, a crude drug obtained from Pistacia lentiscus for gastric and duodenal anti-ulcer activity. *J Ethnopharmacol* 15 (1986): 271–78; Gao, S., and W. Wu. Clinical

and experimental study of *Kuiyangling* in the treatment of chronic superficial gastritis. *Zhong Xi Yi Jie He Za Zhi* 10 (1990): 269–71; Zhang, L., L.W. Yang, and L.J. Yang. Relation between Helicobacter pylori and pathogenesis of chronic atrophic gastritis and the research of its prevention and treatment. *Zhongguo Zhong Xi Yi Jie He Za Zhi* 12 (1992): 521–23; Zhang, X.B., and W. Chen. *Randomized Treatment of 425 Cases of Gastric Ulcer with Kuiyangling Versus Gastridine (Midelid).* Institute of Traditional Chinese Medicine and Pharmacy of Fujian, 1998.

10. Blumenthal, M., A. Goldberg, and J. Brinckmann. *Herbal Medicine: Expanded Commission E Monographs.* Newton, MA: Integrative Medicine Communications, 2000.

11. Ibid.

12. Nitsch, A., and F.P. Nitsch. The clinical use of bovine colostrum. *J Orthomolecular Med* 13 (1998): 110–18; Rona, Z. Bovine colostrum as immune system modulator. *Am J Nat Med* 5.2 (1998): 19–23.

Chapter 10 Chronic Inflammation and Aging

1. Faloon, W. Chronic inflammation. The epidemic disease of aging. *Life Extension* 8 (2002): 13–16.

2. Murray, M.T. *Encyclopedia of Nutritional Supplements.* Rocklin, CA: Prima Publishing, 1996. 239–78.

3. Brandt, K.D. Effects of non-steroidal anti-inflammatory drugs on chondrocyte metabolism *in vitro and in vivo. Am J Med* 83 (1987): 29–34; Brooks, P.M., S.R. Potter, and W.W. Buchanan. NSAID and osteoarthritis—help or hindrance. *J Rheumatol* 9 (1982): 3–5; Newman, N.M., and R.S.M. Ling. Acetabular bone destruction related to non-steroidal anti-inflammatory drugs. *Lancet* 2 (1985): 11–13.

4. McCarthy, D.M. Mechanisms of mucosal injury and healing of non-steroidal anti-inflammatory drugs. *Scan Gastroenterol* suppl. 2080 (1995): 24–29; Jenkins, A.P., D.R. Trew, and B.J. Crump. Do non-steroidal anti-inflammatory drugs increase colonic permeability? *Gut* 32 (1991): 66–69.

5. Murray, *Encyclopedia of Nutritional Supplements.* 336–42.

6. Newmark, T.M., and P. Schulick. *Beyond Aspirin.* Prescott, AZ: Hohm Press, 2000.

7. Ibid.

8. Ibid.

9. Murray, *Encyclopedia of Nutritional Supplements.* 320–31.

10. Pati, K., and A.J. Degidio. *Vitamin & Herbal Digest.* Burlingame, CA: New Editions Publishing, 1996.

11. Murray, Michael T. *The Healing Power of Herbs.* Rocklin, CA: Prima Publishing, 1995.

12. Ibid.

13. Ibid.

Chapter 11 Shields for the Immune System

1. Sanchez, A., et al. Role of sugars in human neutrophilic phagocytosis. *Am J Clin Nutr* 26 (1973): 1180.

2. Kelley, D.S. Modulation of human immune and inflammatory responses by dietary fatty acids. *Nutrition* 17.7–8 (2001): 669–73.

3. Szabo, G. Monocytes, alcohol use, and altered immunity. *Alcohol Clin Exp Res* 22 (1998): 216–19S.

4. Chandra, R.K. Nutrition and the immune system: an introduction. *Am J Clin Nutr* 66 (1997): 460–63S [review].

5. Nieman, D.C. Exercise and resistance to infection. *Can J Physiol Pharmacol* 76 (1998): 573–80 [review].

6. Herbert, T.B., and S. Cohen. Stress and immunity in humans: a meta-analytic review. *Psychosom Med* 55 (1993): 364–79 [review]; Palmblad, J.E. Stress-related modulation of immunity: a review of human studies. *Cancer Detect Prev Suppl* 1 (1987): 57–64 [review].

7. Halley, F.M. Self-regulation of the immune system through biobehavioral strategies. *Biofeedback Self Regul* 16 (1991): 55–74 [review].

8. Kelley, D.S., and A. Bendich. Essential nutrients and immunologic functions. *Am J Clin Nutr* 63.6 (1996): 994S–96S.

9. Glasziou, P.P., and D.E.M. Mackerras. Vitamin A supplementation in infectious diseases: a meta-analysis. *BMJ* 306 (1993): 366–70.

10. Murata, T., et al. Effect of long-term administration of beta-carotene on lymphocyte subsets in humans. *Am J Clin Nutr* 60 (1994): 597–602.

11. Santos, M.S., et al. Natural killer cell activity in elderly men is enhanced by beta-carotene supplementation. *Am J Clin Nutr* 64 (1996): 772–77.

12. Banic, S. Immunostimulation by vitamin C. *Int J Vitam Nutr Res Suppl* 23 (1982): 49–52 [review].

13. Hemilä, H. Vitamin C and the common cold. *Br J Nutr* 67 (1992): 3–16; Hemilä, H. Vitamin C and common cold incidence: a review of studies with subjects under heavy physical stress. *Int J Sports Med* 17 (1996): 379–83.

14. Meydani, S.N., et al. Vitamin E supplementation enhances cell-mediated immunity in healthy elderly subjects. *Am J Clin Nutr* 52 (1990): 557–63; Penn, N.D., et al. The effect of dietary supplementation with vitamins A, C and E on cell-mediated immune function in elderly long-stay patients: a randomized controlled trial. *Age Ageing* 20 (1991): 169–74.

15. Kim, J.M., and R.H. White. Effect of vitamin E on the anticoagulant response to warfarin. *Am J Cardiol* 77 (1996): 545–46.

16. Tamura, J., et al. Immunomodulation by vitamin B12: augmentation of CD8+ T lymphocytes and natural killer (NK) cell activity in vitamin B12-deficient patients by methyl-B12 treatment. *Clin Exp Immunol* 116 (1999): 28–32.

17. Snow, C.F. Laboratory diagnosis of vitamin B12 and folate deficiency. A guide for the primary care physician. *Arch Intern Med* 159 (1999): 1289–98 [review].

18. Fraker, P.J., et al. Interrelationships between zinc and immune function. *Fed Proc* 45 (1986): 1474–79; Macknin, M.L. Zinc lozenges for the common cold. *Cleveland Clin J Med* 66 (1999): 27–32 [review].

19. Chandra, R.K. Excessive intake of zinc impairs immune responses. *JAMA* 252 (1984): 1443–46.

20. Scaglione, F., et al. Immunomodulatory effects of two extracts of *Panax ginseng* CA Meyer. *Drugs Exptl Clin Res* 16 (1990): 537–42.

21. See, D.M., et al. In vitro effects of echinacea and ginseng on natural killer and antibody-dependent cell cytotoxicity in healthy subjects and chronic fatigue syndrome or acquired immunodeficiency

syndrome patients. *Immunopharmacology* 35 (1997): 229–35; Melchart, D., et al. Immunomodulation with echinacea—a systematic review of controlled clinical trials. *Phytomed* 1 (1994): 245–54.

22. Melchart.

23. Melchart, D., et al. Echinacea root extracts for the prevention of upper respiratory tract infections: a double-blind, placebo-controlled randomized trial. *Arch Fam Med* 7 (1998): 541–45.

24. Bengmark, S. Immunonutrition: role of biosurfactants, fiber, and probiotic bacteria. *Nutrition* 14 (1998): 585–94 [review].

25. Rasic, J.L. The role of dairy foods containing bifido and acidophilus bacteria in nutrition and health. *N Eur Dairy J* 4 (1983): 80–88; Barefoot, S.F., and T.R. Klaenhammer. Detection and activity of Lactacin B, a Bacteriocin produced by Lactobacillus acidophilus. *Appl Environ Microbiol* 45 (1983): 1808–15.

26. Fiocchi, A., et al. A double-blind clinical trial for the evaluation of the therapeutic effectiveness of a calf thymus derivative (Thymomodulin) in children with recurrent respiratory infections. *Thymus* 8 (1986): 831–39; Vettori, G., et al. Prevention of recurrent respiratory infections in adults. *Minerva Med* 78 (1987): 1281–89.

27. Garagiola, U., M. Buzzetti, and E. Cardella. Immunological patterns during regular intensive training in athletes: quantification and evaluation of a preventive pharmacological approach. *J Int Med Res* 23 (1995): 85–95; Wysocki, J., et al. The influence of thymus extracts on the chemotaxis of polymorphonuclear neutrophils (PMN) from patients with insulin-dependent diabetes mellitus (IDD). *Thymus* 20 (1992): 63–67.

28. Immunesupport.com. "Studies Show Oil of Oregano Fights Bacterial Infections" 10 June 2002 <www.immunesupport.com/library/showarticle.cfm/id/3178>.

Chapter 12 Fight Fat and Win!

1. *JAMA* 286.10 (12 Sept. 2001): 1195–1200.

2. Health Canada. 1990 National Population Health Survey. Canadian Community Health Survey 2000/2001.

3. U.S. Congress. *Deception and Fraud in the Diet Industry, Part 1.* Washington, DC: Government Printing Office, 1990. 101–50.

4. National Institutes of Health. Consensus conference on methods for voluntary weight loss and control. *Ann Int Med* 116 (1992): 942–49; Kramer, F.M., et al. Long-term follow-up of behavioural treatment of obesity: patterns of regain among men and women. *Intl J Obesiy* 13 (1989): 123–26.

5. World Health Organization. *Obesity: Preventing and Managing the Global Epidemic.* Report of a WHO Consultation on Obesity. Geneva: WHO, 1998.

6. *Report of the Task Force on the Treatment of Obesity.* Ottawa, ON: Minister of Supplies and Services Canada, 1991; Manson, J.E., et al. Body weight and mortality. *N Engl J Med* 333 (1995): 677–85.

7. Lean, M.E., et al. Waist circumference as a measure for indicating need for weight management. *BMJ* 311 (1995): 158–61.

8. National Institute of Diabetes and Digestive and Kidney Diseases. *Understanding Adult Obesity.* Rockville, MD: National Institutes of Health, 1993.

9. King, B.J. *Fat Wars.* Toronto: Macmillan Canada, 2000. 9.

10. Kandulska, K., L. Nogowski, and T. Szkudelski. Effect of some phytoestrogens on metabolism of rat adipocytes. *Reprod Nutr Dev* 39 (1999): 497–501.

11. Adlercreutz, H., et al. Inhibition of human aromatase by mammalian lignans and isoflavonoid phytoestrogens. *J Steroid Biochem Molec Biol* 44.2 (1993): 147–53.

12. Colker, C.M., et al. Effects of citrus aurantium extract, caffeine, and St. John's wort on body fat loss, lipid levels, and mood states in overweight healthy adults. *Curr Ther Res* 60 (1999): 145–53.

13. MacDonald, H.B. Conjugated linoleic acid and disease prevention: a review of current knowledge. *J Am Coll* 19.2 (2000): 111S–118S.

14. Kaats, G.R., et al. Effects of chromium picolinate supplementation on body composition: a randomized, double-masked, placebo-controlled study. *Curr Ther Res* 57 (1996): 747–56.

15. Dulloo, A.G., et al. Efficacy of a green tea extract rich in catechin polyphenols and caffeine in increasing 24-h energy expenditure and fat oxidation in humans. *Am J Clin Nutr* 70 (1999): 1040–45.

16. Ballerini, R. Evaluation of efficacy and safety of a food supplement for weight control through the reduced calories-intake from carbohydrates vs. placebo. Data on file. Pharmachem Laboratories, Kearny, NJ, 2002.

17. King. *Fat Wars*. 78.

Chapter 13 Osteoporosis: Outwitting the Silent Thief

1. National Institutes of Health, Osteoporosis and Related Bone Diseases—National Resource Centre. "Fact Sheets—Osteoporosis Overview" <www.osteo.org>. National Institutes of Health, Osteoporosis and Related Bone Diseases—National Resource Centre. 3 June 2002 <www.osteo.org/newfile.asp?doc=osteo&doctitle=Osteoporosis+Overview&doctype= HTML+Fact+Sheet>.

2. Osteoporosis Society of Canada. "What is Osteoporosis?" <www.osteoporosis.ca>. Osteoporosis Society of Canada. 3 June 2002 <www.osteoporosis.ca/OSTEO/D01-01.html>.

3. National Institute of Arthritis and Musculoskeletal and Skin Diseases, "Osteoporosis: Progress and Promise" <www.niams.nih.gov>. National Institute of Arthritis and Musculoskeletal and Skin Diseases, National Institutes of Health. 3 June 2002 <http://www.niams.nih.gov/hi/topics/osteoporosis/opbkgr.htm>.

4. National Institutes of Health. Consensus Statement Online. "Optimal Calcium Intake." 12.4 (6–8 1994 June): 1-31. <www.nih.gov>. 3 June 2002 <odp.od.nih.gov/consensus/cons/097/097_statement.htm>.

5. National Institutes of Health, Osteoporosis and Related Bone Diseases—National Resource Centre. "Fact Sheets—Osteoporosis Overview" <www.osteo.org>. National Institutes of Health, Osteoporosis and Related Bone Diseases—National Resource Centre. 3 June 2002 <www.osteo.org/newfile.asp?doc=osteo&doctitle=Osteoporosis+Overview&doctype= HTML+Fact+Sheet>.

6. Standing Committee on the Scientific Evaluation of Dietary Reference Intakes, Food and Nutrition Board, Institute of Medicine. *Dietary Reference Intakes for Calcium, Phosphorus, Magnesium, Vitamin D, and Fluoride*. Washington DC: National Academy Press, 1997.

7. Ibid.

8. Osteoporosis Society of Canada. "Prevention—Calcium & Vitamin D: An Essential Element for Bone Health" <www.osteoporosis.ca>. Osteoporosis Society of Canada. 3 June 2002 < www.osteoporosis.ca/OSTEO/D02-01d.html#vitamind>.

9. Messina, M.J. Legumes and soybeans: overview of their nutritional profiles and health effects. *Am J Clin Nutr* 70 (1999): 439S–450S.

10. Somekawa, Y., et al. Soy intake related to menopause symptoms, serum lipids, and bone mineral density in postmenopausal Japanese women. *Obstet Gynecol* 97 (2001): 109–115.

11. van Papendorp, D.H., H. Coetzer, and M.C. Kruger. Biochemical profile of osteoporotic patients on essential fatty acid supplementation. *Nutr Res* 15 (1995): 325–34.

12. Kruger, M.C., et al. Calcium, gamma-linolenic acid and eicosapentaenoic acid supplementation in senile osteoporosis. *Aging* 10 (1998): 385–94.

13. Osteoporosis Society of Canada. "Prevention—Calcium & Vitamin D: An Essential Element for Bone Health" <www.osteoporosis.ca>. Osteoporosis Society of Canada. 3 June 2002 <www.osteoporosis.ca/OSTEO/D02-01c.html>.

14. Kerstetter, J.E., and L.H. Allen. Dietary protein increases urinary calcium. *J Nutr* 120 (1990): 134–36.

15. Feskanich, D., et al. Protein consumption and bone fractures in women. *Am J Epidemiol* 143 (1996): 472–79.

16. Abelow, B.J., T.R. Holford, and K.L. Insogna. Cross-cultural associations between dietary animal protein and hip fracture: a hypothesis. *Calcif Tissue Int* 50 (1992): 14–18.

17. Wyshak, G., and R.E. Frisch. Carbonated beverages, dietary calcium, the dietary calcium/phosphorus ratio, and bone fractures in girls and boys. *J Adolesc Health* 15 (1994): 210–15.

18. Mazariegos-Ramos, E., et al. Consumption of soft drinks with phosphoric acid as a risk factor for the development of hypocalcemia in children: a case-control study. *J Pediatr* 126 (1995): 940–42.

19. Cohen, L., and R. Kitzes. Infrared spectroscopy and magnesium content of bone mineral in osteoporotic women. *Israeli Journal of Medical Science* 17 (1981): 1123–25; Geinster, J.Y., et al. Preliminary report of decreased serum magnesium in postmenopausal osteoporosis. *Magnesium* 8 (1989): 106–9; Cohen, L., A. Laor, and R. Kitzes. Magnesium malabsorption in postmenopausal osteoporosis. *Magnesium* 2 (1983): 139–43.

20. Dimai, H-P., et al. Daily oral magnesium supplementation suppresses bone turnover in young adult males. *J Clin Endocrinol Metab* 83 (1998): 2742–8; Stendig-Lindberg, G., R. Tepper, and I. Leichter. Trabecular bone density in a two year controlled trial of peroral magnesium in osteoporosis. *Magnesium Research* 6 (1993): 155–63.

21. Eisinger, J., and D. Clairet. Effects of silicon, fluoride, etidronate and magnesium on bone mineral density: a retrospective study. *Magnesium Research* 6 (1993): 247–49.

22. Head, K.A. Ipriflavone: an important bone-building isoflavone. *Altern Med Rev* 4 (1999): 10–22 [review]; Adami, S., et al. Ipriflavone prevents radial bone loss in postmenopausal women with low bone mass over 2 years. *Osteoporos Int* 7.2 (1997): 119–25; Gennari, C., et al. Effect of ipriflavone—a synthetic derivative of natural isoflavones—on bone mass loss in the early years after menopause. *Menopause* 5.1 (1998): 9–15.

23. Osteoporosis Society of Canada. "Treatment: The Role of Hormone Therapy in the Prevention and Treatment of Osteoporosis" <www.osteoporosis.ca>. Osteoporosis Society of Canada. 3 June 2002 <www.osteoporosis.ca/OSTEO/D04-01e.html>.

24. Ettinger, B., et al. Reduction of vertebral fracture risk in postmenopausal women with osteoporosis treated with raloxifene. *JAMA* 282 (1999): 637–45.

25. Osteoporosis Society of Canada. "Treatment: Bisphosphonates, an Option for the Prevention and Treatment of Osteoporosis" <www.osteoporosis.ca>. Osteoporosis Society of Canada. 3 June 2002 <www.osteoporosis.ca/OSTEO/D04-01-02.html>.

Chapter 14 See Me, Hear Me

1. Prevent Blindness America. "Vision Problems in the U.S.: Prevalence of Adult Visual Impairment and Age-Related Eye Disease, National Institutes of Health, National Eye Institute. 15 March 2002 <www.preventblindness.org/vpus/cataract.pdf>.

2. The Lighthouse. *The Lighthouse National Survey on Vision Loss: The Experience, Attitudes and Knowledge of Middle-Aged and Older Americans.* New York: The Lighthouse, Louis Harris and Associates, 1994.

3. Alliance for Eye and Vision Research. "A Vision of Hope for Older Americans' Progress and Opportunities in Eye and Vision Research." An official report to the White House Conference on Aging, 1995.

4. Prevent Blindness America. "Vision Problems in the U.S."

5. Ringsdorf, W.M. Jr., and E. Cheraskin. Ascorbic acid and glaucoma: a review. *J Holistic Med* 3 (1981): 67–72.

6. Gaspar, A.Z., P. Gasser, and J. Flammer. The influence of magnesium on visual field and peripheral vasospasm in glaucoma. *Ophthalmologica* 209 (1995): 11–13; Filina, A.A., et al. Lipoic acid as a means of metabolic therapy of open-angle glaucoma. *Vestn Oftalmol* 111 (1995): 6–8.

7. Prevent Blindness America. "Vision Problems in the U.S."

8. Kahn, H.A., et al. "The Framingham Eye Study. I. Outline and major prevalence findings." *Am J Epidemiol* 106 (1977): 17–32; Klein, B.E., R. Klein, and K.L. Linton. Prevalence of age-related lens opacities in a population: the Beaver Dam Eye Study." *Ophthalmol* 99 (1002): 546–52.

9. West, S.K., and C.T. Valmadrid. Epidemiology of risk factors for age-related cataract. *Surg Ophthalmol* 39.4 (1995): 323–34.

10. Kupfer, C. NEI, NIH. The conquest of cataract: a global challenge. *Trans Ophthalmol* S UK 1984: 1041–10.

11. Eye Disease Case-Control Study Group. Antioxidant status and neovascular age-related macular degeneration. *Arch Ophthalmol* 111 (1993): 104–9; Seddon, J.M., et al. Dietary carotenoids, vitamins A, C, and E, and advanced age-related macular degeneration. *JAMA* 272 (1994): 1413–20.

12. Chasen-Taber, L., et al. A prospective study of carotenoid and vitamin A intakes and risk of cataract extraction in US women. *Am J Clin Nutr* 70 (1999): 509–16.

13. Gray-Donald, K. "Lutein, zeaxanthin and lycopene intakes among Canadian adults." Montreal, PQ: McGill University, 2000.

14. Sala, D., et al. Effect of anthocyanosides on visual performance at low illumination. *Minerva Oftalmol* 21 (1979): 283–85.

15. Mian, E., et al. Anthocyanosides and the walls of microvessels: further aspects of the mechanism of action of their protective in syndromes due to abnormal capillary fragility. *Minerva Med* 68 (1977): 3565–81.

16. Ibid.; Jacques, P.F., and L.T. Chylack Jr. Epidemiologic evidence of a role for the antioxidant vitamins and carotenoids in cataract prevention. *Am J Clin Nutr* 53 (1991): 352S–55S; Jacques, P.F., et al. Antioxidant status in persons with and without senile cataract. *Arch Ophthalmol* 106 (1988): 337–40.

17. Ringsdorf. Ascorbic acid.

18. Gisnger, C., et al. Effect of vitamin E supplementation on platelet thromboxane A2 production in type I diabetic patients: double-blind crossover trial. *Diabetes* 37 (1988): 1260–64.

19. Ross, W.M., et al. Modelling cortical cataractogenesis: 3. In vivo effects of vitamin E on cataractogenesis in diabetic rats. *Can J Ophthalmol* 17 (1982): 61.

20. Lanthony, P., and J.P. Cosson. Evolution of color vision in diabetic retinopathy treated by extract of *Ginkgo biloba. J Fr Ophthalmol* 11 (1988): 671–74.

21. Lebuisson, D.A., L. Leroy, and G. Reigal. Treatment of senile macular degeneration with *Ginkgo biloba* extract: a preliminary double-blind study versus placebo. In *Rokan (Ginkgo biloba): Recent Results in Pharmacology and Clinic,* edited by F.W. Fünfgeld. Berlin: Springer-Verlag, 1988. 231–36.

22. Lanthony and Cosson. Evolution of color vision.

23. Desai, M., et al. "Trends in Vision and Hearing Among Older Americans." <cdc.gov/nchs>. National Center for Health Statistics. 20 March 2002 <www.cdc.gov/nchs/data/agingtrends/02vision.pdf>.

24. Ries, P.W. Prevalence and characteristics of persons with hearing trouble. *Vital and Health Statistics* 10.188 (1994): 5–8.

25. Hearing Education and Awareness for Rockers. 20 March 2002 <www.hearnet.com>.

26. Ruth, R.A., and R. Hamill-Ruth. A multidisciplinary approach to management of tinnutis and hyperacusis. *The Hearing Journal* 54.11 (2001): 26.

27. "Tinnitus: Noise 24 hours a day" <hear-it.org>. hear-it AISBL. 14 March 2002 <www.hear-it.org/page.pl?page=1530>.

28. Florida Ear and Sinus Center, "Ear Research Publication Summaries: Effect of melatonin on tinnitus" <www.ear-sinusctr.com>. 20 March 2002 <www.ear-sinusctr.com/summaries.html>.

29. Mayo Foundation for Medical Education and Research, "Ginkgo, Adapted from *Your Guide to Herbal Supplement*" <www.mayoclinic.com>. MayoClinic.com. 20 March 2002 <www.mayoclinic.com/findinformation/conditioncenters/invoke.cfm?objectid=FE319FC4-1A54-4E5C-B15A48A74FB7F06A>.

30. Mayo Foundation for Medical Education and Research, "Vitamin B-12 (cobalamin)" <www.mayoclinic.com>. MayoClinic.com. 20 March 2002 <www.mayoclinic.com/findinformation/healthylivingcenter/invoke.cfm?objectid=4F07C6A1-A35D-4D12-B695DD05A01745DE>.

31. Canadian Hearing Society. *Get Connected to Facts on Tinnutis: A Guide for Tinnutis Sufferers and Their Doctors.* Toronto, 2001.

32. Cruickshanks, K.J., et al. Cigarette smoking and hearing loss: the Epidemiology of Hearing Loss Study. *JAMA* 279.21 (1998): 1715–19.

Chapter 15 Women's Health: Menopause and Beyond

1. Raz, R., and W. Stamm. A controlled trial of intravaginal estriol in postmenopausal women with recurrent urinary tract infections. *N Engl J Med* 329 (1993): 753–56.

2. Henderson, V.W. Estrogen, cognition and a woman's risk of Alzheimer's disease. *Am J Med* 103 (1997): 115–85.

3. Grodstein, F., P.A. Newcomb, and M.J. Stampfer. Postmenopausal hormone therapy and the risk of colo-rectal cancer: a review and meta-analysis. *Am J Med* 106 (1999): 574–82.

4. Risks and benefits of estrogen plus progestin in healthy postmenopausal women: principal results from the Women's Health Initiative randomized controlled trial. *JAMA* 288.3 (2002): 321–33, 366–68.

5. Campagnoli, C., et al. HRT and breast cancer risk: a clue for interpreting the available data. *Maturitas* 33 (1999): 185–90.

6. Risks and benefits of estrogen plus progestin in healthy postmenopausal women: principal results from the Women's Health Initiative randomized controlled trial. *JAMA* 288.3 (2002): 321–33, 366–68.; Grady, D., et al. Cardiovascular disease outcomes during 6.8 years of hormone therapy. Heart and estrogen/progestin replacement follow-up study (HERS II) *JAMA* 288.1 (2002): 49–57.

7. Grady, D., et al. Cardiovascular disease outcomes during 6.8 years of hormone therapy. Heart and estrogen/progestin replacement follow-up study (HERS II) *JAMA* 288.1 (2002): 49–57, 58–66, 99–101.

8. Recker, R.R., et al. The effect of low-dose continuous estrogen and progesterone therapy with calcium and vitamin D on bone in elderly women. A randomized, controlled trial. *Ann Intern Med* 130.ll (1 June 1999): 897–904.

9. Stampfer, M.J., et al. Vitamin E consumption and the risk of coronary heart disease in women. *N Engl J Med* 328 (1993): 1444–49.

10. Düker, E.M., et al. Effects of extracts from *Cimicifuga racemosa* on gonadotropin release in menopausal women and ovariectomized rats. *Planta Medica* 57 (1991): 420–44.

11. Bone, K. *Vitex agnus-castus:* Scientific studies and clinical applications. *Eur J Herbal Med* 1 (1994): 12–15.

12. Le Bars, P.L., et al. A placebo-controlled, double-blind, randomized trial of an extract of *Ginkgo biloba* for dementia. North American EGb Study Group. *JAMA* 278 (1997): 1327–32.

13. Nestel, P.J., et al. Isoflavones from red clover improve systemic arterial compliance but not plasma lipids in menopausal women. *J Clin Endocrinol Metab* 84 (1999): 895–98.

14. Woelk, H. Comparison of St. John's wort and imipramine for treating depression: randomized controlled trial. *BMJ* 321 (2000): 536–39; Philipp, M., R. Kohnen, and K.O. Hiller. Hypericum extract versus imipramine or placebo in patients with moderate depression: randomized multicenter study of treatment for eight weeks. *BMJ* 319 (1999):1534–39.

15. Leathwood, P.D., et al. Aqueous extract of valerian root (*Valeriana officinalis* L) improves sleep quality in man. *Pharmacol Biochem Behav* 17 (1982): 65–71.

16. Araghiniknam, M., et al. Antioxidant activity of dioscorea and dehydroepiandrosterone (DHEA) in older humans. *Life Sci* 11 (1996): 147–57.

17. Anderson, J.W., B.M. Johnstone, and M.E. Cook-Newell. Meta-analysis of the effects of soy protein intake on serum lipids. *N Engl J Med* 333 (1995): 276–82; Albertazzi, P., et al. The effect of dietary soy supplementation on hot flushes. *Obstet Gynecol* 91 (1998): 6–11; Potter, S.M., et al. Soy protein and isoflavones: their effects on blood lipids and bone density in postmenopausal women. *Am J Clin Nutr* 68, suppl. (1998): 1375S–79S.

18. Cave, W.T., Jr. Dietary n-3 (omega-3) polyunsaturated fatty acid effects on animal tumorigenesis. *FASEB J* 5 (1991): 2160–66 [review].

19. Slaven, L., and C. Lee. Mood and symptom reporting among middle-aged women: the relationship between menopausal status, hormone replacement therapy, and exercise participation. *Health Psychol* 16 (1997): 203–8.

Chapter 16 Men's Health: Functioning South of the Border

1. Arrighi, H.M., et al. Natural history of benign prostatic hyperplasia and risk of prostatectomy: the Baltimore Longitudinal Study of Aging. *Urology* 38, suppl. (1991).

2. Horton, R. Benign prostatic hyperplasia: a disorder of androgen metabolism in the male. *J Am Geri Soc* 32 (1984): 380–85.

3. Suzuki, K., et al. Endocrine environment of benign prostatic hyperplasia: prostate size and volume are correlated with serum estrogen concentration. *Scand J Urol Nephrol* 29 (March 1995): 65–68; Farnsworth, W.E. Roles of estrogen and SHBG in prostate physiology. *Prostate* 28 (1996): 17–23; Stone, N.N., et al. Aromatization of androstenedione to estrogen by benign prostatic secretions. *Urol Res* 15 (1987): 165–67; Ekman, P., et al. Estrogen receptors in human prostate: evidence for multiple binding sites. *J Clin Endocrinol Metab* 57 (1983): 166–76; Hiramatsu, M., et al. Aromatase in hyperplasia and carcinoma of the human prostate. *Prostate* 31 (1997): 118–24.

4. Colborn, T., D. Dumanoski, and J. Peterson Myers. *Our Stolen Future*. New York: Penguin Books, 1996.

5. Gordon, G.D., et al. Conversion of androgens to estrogens in cirrhosis of the liver. *J Clin Endocrinol Metab* 40 (1975): 1018–26; Willis, B.R., et al. Ethanol-induced male reproductive tract pathology as a function of ethanol dose and duration of exposure. *J Pharmacol Exp Therapeu* 225 (1983): 470–78; Kappas, A., et al. Nutrition-endocrine interactions: induction of reciprocal changes in the delta-5-alpha-reduction of testosterone and the cytochrome P-450-dependent oxidation of estradiol by dietary macronutrients in man. *Proc Natl Acad Sci USA* 80 (1083): 7646–49; Chyou, P.H., et al. A prospective study of alcohol, diet, and other lifestyle factors in relation to obstructive uropathy. *Prostate* 22 (1993): 253–64.

6. Prasad, A.S. Zinc status and serum testosterone levels on healthy adults. *Nutr* 12 (1996): 344–48; Hunt, C.D., et al. Effects of dietary zinc depletion on seminal volume and zinc loss, serum testosterone concentrations, and sperm morphology in young men. *Am J Clin Nutr* 56 (1992): 148–57.

7. Kappas, Nutrition-endocrine interactions.

8. Simon, D., et al. Interrelation between plasma testosterone and plasma insulin in healthy adult men: the Telecom Study. *Diabetologia* 35 (1992): 173–77.

9. Blumenthal, M., A. Goldberg, and J. Brinckmann. *Herbal Medicine*. Expanded Commission E Monographs. Newton, MA: Integrative Medicine Communications, 2000.

10. Ibid.

11. Murray, M.T. *The Healing Power of Herbs*. Rocklin, CA: Prima Publishing, 1995.

12. Rae, M. Saw palmetto doesn't work! Defined pollen extract for prostate health. *The Holistic Lifestyle* Sept. 2000: 1–8.

13. Holt, S. *Soya for Health: The Definitive Medical Guide.* Larchmont, NY: Mary Ann Liebert, 1996.

14. Hall, D.C. Nutritional influences on estrogen metabolism. *Applied Nutritional Science Reports.* MET451. San Clemente, CA, 2001.

15. Hobbs, C. Medicinal Mushrooms: An Exploration of Tradition, Healing and Culture. Santa Cruz, CA: Botanica Press, 1995.

Chapter 17 Keeping Your Marbles

1. Perls, T., and M. Hutter Silver. *Living to 100.* New York: Basic Books, 1999; Goldman, D. *Emotional Intelligence: Why It Can Matter More Than IQ.* New York: Bantam Books, 1995.

2. Blaylock, R. *Excitotoxins: The Taste That Kills.* Santa Fe, NM: Health Press, 1997.

3. Perls, *Living to 100.*

4. Cherniske, S. *Caffeine Blues: Wake Up to the Hidden Dangers of America's #1 Drug.* New York: Warner. 1998.

5. Wassef, F. Pharmacological ramifications of grains. *International Journal of Integrative Medicine* Jan./Feb. 2001: 6–11.

6. Mattson, M.P. Neuroplasticity and how the brain adapts to aging. *Geriatrics & Aging* 4 (2001): 24–25.

7. Perrig, W.J., P. Perrig, and H.B. Stahelin. The relation between antioxidants and memory performance in the old and very old. *J Am Geriatr Soc* 45 (1997): 718–24; Ortega, R.M., et al. Dietary intake and cognitive function in a group of elderly people. *Am J Clin Nutr* 66 (1997): 803–9.

8. Rae, M. Methylcobalamin: armour for your nervous system. *The Holistic Lifestyle* May 2001.

9. Lebars, P.L., et al. A placebo-controlled, double-blind, randomized trial of an extract of ginkgo biloba for dementia. *JAMA* 278 (1997): 1327–32.

10. Secades, J.J., and G. Frontera. CDP-choline: pharmaceutical and clinical review. *Methods Find Exp Clin Pharmacol* 17 (1995): 2–54; Spiers, P.A., et al. Citicoline improves verbal memory in aging. *Arch Neurol* 53 (1996): 411–48; Alvarez, A.X., et al. Citicoline improves memory performance in elderly subjects. *Methods Find Exp Clin Pharmacol* 19 (1997): 201–10.

11. Murray, M. *Encyclopedia of Nutritional Supplements.* Rocklin, CA: Prima Publishing, 1996.

12. Kidd, P.M. *Phosphatidylserine (PS): A Remarkable Brain Cell Nutrient.* Decatur, IL: Lucas Meyer, 1998.

13. Cloister, D. *SAM-e: What You Need to Know.* Garden City Park, NY: Avery Publishing, 1999.

14. Murray M. *The Healing Power of Herbs.* Rocklin, CA: Prima Publishing, 1995.

15. Ibid.

Chapter 18 Heart Disease: Following a New Beat

1. American Heart Association, Cardiovascular Disease Statistics <www.americanheart.org> 26 March 2002 <216.185.112.5/presenter.jhtml?identifier=4478>; Heart and Stroke Foundation of Canada. "Prevention—Tips to reduce your risk of heart disease." <ww2.heartandstroke.ca>. Heart and

Stroke Foundation of Canada. 22 March 2002 <ww2.heartandstroke.ca/Page.asp?PageID=110&ArticleID=588&Src=heart>.

2. American Heart Association. "Cardiovascular Disease Statistics" <www.americanheart.org>. American Heart Association. 26 March 2002 <216.185.112.5/presenter.jhtml?identifier=4478>.

3. Heart and Stroke Foundation of Canada. 21 Oct. 2002 <ww1.heartandstroke.ca/Page.asp?PageID=33&ArticleID=581&Src=heart&From=SubCategory>.

4. Health Canada. *Canadians and Heart Health: Reducing the Risk.* Ministry of Supply and Services Canada, Cat. H39-328/1995E, Ottawa, 1995. 7.

5. Heart and Stroke Foundation of Canada. "Risk Factors – Smoking" <ww2.heartandstroke.ca>. Heart and Stroke Association of Canada. 22 March 2002 <ww2.heartandstroke.ca/Page.asp?PageID=33&ArticleID=594&Src=heart&From=SubCategory>.

6. Health Canada. *Canadians and Heart Health: Reducing the Risk.* Ministry of Supply and Services Canada, Cat. H39-328/1995E. Ottawa, 1995. 9.

7. Health Canada. *Canadians and Heart Health.* 7; Shekelle, R.B., and J. Stamler. Dietary cholesterol and ischaemic heart disease. *Lancet* 1 (1989): 1177–79.

8. Health Canada. *Canadians and Heart Health.* 9.

9. National Academy on an Aging Society. *Challenges for the 21st Century: Chronic and Disabling Conditions.* No. 12. Washington, DC, Oct. 2000. 3.

10. Heart and Stroke Foundation of Canada. "Prevention—Tips to reduce your risk of heart disease" <ww2.heartandstroke.ca>. Heart and Stroke Foundation of Canada. 22 March 2002 <ww2.heartandstroke.ca/Page.asp?PageID=110&ArticleID=588&Src=heart>.

11. Wassef, F. "Cardiovascular disease: reading the correct road signs. *Am J Natural Med* 5.7 (Sept. 1998).

12. American Heart Association. "Tests to Diagnose Heart Disease" <www.americanheart.org>. American Heart Association. 28 March 2002 <www.americanheart.org/presenter.jhtml?identifier=4739>.

13. Ibid.

14. National Institutes of Health. "NIH Consensus Statement Online" <www.nih.gov>, 13.3:1–33. 29 March 2002 <consensus.nih.gov/cons/101/101_statement.htm>.

15. Ibid.

16. Lee, I-M. et al. Physical activity and coronary heart disease in women: is "no pain, no gain" passé? *JAMA* 285 (2001): 1447–54.

17. Lee, I-M., H.D. Sesso, and R.S. Paffenbarger, Jr. Physical activity and coronary heart disease risk in men: does the duration of exercise episodes predict risk? *Circulation* 102 (2000): 981–86.

18. National Institutes of Health. "NIH Consensus Statement Online" <www.nih.gov>, 13.3:1–33. 29 March 2002 <consensus.nih.gov/cons/101/101_statement.htm>.

19. Morris, M.C., F. Sacks, and B. Rosner. Does fish oil lower blood pressure? A meta-analysis of controlled trials. *Circulation* 88 (1993): 523–33; Von Schacky, C., et al. The effect of dietary omega-3 fatty acids on coronary atherosclerosis: a randomized double-blind, placebo-controlled trial. *Ann Intern Med* 130 (1999): 554–62.

20. Singh, R.B., et al. Randomized, double-blind, placebo-controlled trial of fish oil and mustard oil in patients with suspected acute myocardial infarction: the Indian experiment of infarct survival-4. *Cardiovasc Drugs* 11 (1997): 485–91.

21. Kono, S., et al. Green tea consumption and serum lipid profiles: a cross-sectional study in Northern Kyushu, Japan. *Prev Med* 21 (1992): 526–31; Stensvold, I., et al. Tea consumption: relationship to cholesterol, blood pressure, and coronary and total mortality. *Prev Med* 21 (1992): 546–53; Tsubono, Y., and S. Tsugane. Green tea intake in relation to serum lipid levels in middle-aged Japanese men and women. *Ann Epidemiol* 7 (1997): 280–84.

22. Stampfer, M.J., et al. Vitamin E consumption and the risk of coronary disease in women. *N Engl J Med* 328 (1993): 1444–49; Rimm, E.B., et al. Vitamin E consumption and the risk of coronary heart disease in men. *N Engl J Med* 328 (1993): 1450–56; Stephens, N.G., et al. Randomised controlled trial of vitamin E in patients with coronary disease: Cambridge Heart Antioxidant Study (CHAOS). *Lancet* 347 (1996): 781–86; [No authors listed]. Dietary supplementation with n-3 polyunsaturated fatty acids and vitamin E after myocardial infarction: results of the GISSI-Prevenzione trial. *Lancet* 354 (1999): 447–55.

23. Yusuf, S., et al. Vitamin E supplementation and cardiovascular events in high-risk patients. The Heart Outcomes Prevention Evaluation Study Investigators. *N Engl J Med* 342 (2000): 154–60.

24. Simon, J.A. Vitamin C and cardiovascular disease: a review. *J Am Coll Nutr* 11 (1992): 107–27.

25. Solzbach, U., et al. Vitamin C improves endothelial dysfunction of epicardial coronary arteries in hypertensive patients. *Circulation* 16 (1997): 1513–19.

26. Ness, A.R., D. Chee, and P. Elliott. Vitamin C and blood pressure—an overview. *J Human Hypertens* 11 (1997): 343–50.

27. Balz, F. "Antioxidant Vitamins and Heart Disease." Paper presented at the 60th Annual Biology Colloquium, Oregon State University, 25 Feb. 1999.

28. Singh, R.B., et al. Plasma levels of antioxidant vitamins and oxidative stress in patients with acute myocardial infarction. *Acta Cardiol* 49 (1994): 441–52.

29. Singh, R.B., et al. Usefulness of antioxidant vitamins in suspected acute myocardial infarction (the Indian experiment of infarct survival-3). *Am J Cardiol* 77 (1996): 232–36.

30. Head, K.A. Inositol hexaniacinate: a safer alternative to niacin. *Alt Med Rev* 1 (1996): 176–84 [review].

31. Murray, M. Lipid-lowering drugs vs. Inositol hexaniacinate. *Am J Natural Med* 2 (1995): 9–12 [review].

32. Ubbink, J.B., et al. Vitamin requirements for the treatment of hyperhomocysteinemia in humans. *J Nutr* 124 (1994): 1927–33.

33. Griffith, L.E., et al. The influence of dietary and nondietary calcium supplementation on blood pressure: an updated metaanalysis of randomized controlled trials. *Am J Hypertens* 12 (1999): 84–92.

34. Bell, L., et al. Cholesterol-lowering effects of calcium carbonate in patients with mild to moderate hypercholesterolemia. *Arch Intern Med* 152 (1992): 2441–44; Bostick, R.M., et al. Effect of calcium supplementation on serum cholesterol and blood pressure: a randomized, double-blind, placebo-controlled, clinical trial. *Arch Fam Med* 9 (2000): 31–39.

35. Nozue, T., et al. Magnesium status, serum HDL cholesterol, and apolipoprotein A-1 levels. *J Pediatr Gastroenterol Nutr* 20 (1995): 316–18; Davis, W.H., et al. Monotherapy with magnesium increases

abnormally low high density lipoprotein cholesterol: a clinical assay. *Curr Ther Res* 36 (1984): 341–46.

36. Motoyama, T., et al. Oral magnesium supplementation in patients with essential hypertension. *Hypertension* 13 (1989): 227–32.

37. Dyckner, T., and P.O. Wester. Effect of magnesium on blood pressure. *BMJ* 286 (1983): 1847–49.

38. Oster, O., et al. The serum selenium concentration of patients with acute myocardial infarction. *Ann Clin Res* 18 (1986): 36–42; Korpela, H., et al. Effect of selenium supplementation after acute myocardial infarction. *Res Commun Chem Pathol Pharmacol* 65 (1989): 249–52.

39. Beaglehole, R., et al. Decreased blood selenium and risk of myocardial infarction. *Int J Epidemiol* 19 (1990): 918–22.

40. Kuklinski, B., E. Weissenbacher, and A. Fahnrich. Coenzyme Q10 and antioxidants in acute myocardial infarction. *Mol Aspects Med* 15, suppl. (1994): S143–S147.

41. Langsjoen, P., et al. Treatment of essential hypertension with coenzyme Q10. *Mol Aspects Med* 15, suppl. (1994): S265–S272.; Digiesi, V., F. Cantini, and B. Brodbeck. Effect of coenzyme Q10 on essential arterial hypertension. *Curr Ther Res* 47 (1990): 841–45; Singh, R.B., et al. Effect of hydrosoluble coenzyme Q10 on blood pressures and insulin resistance in hypertensive patients with coronary artery disease. *J Hum Hypertens* 13 (1999): 203–8.

42. Singh, R.B., and M.A. Niaz. Serum concentration of lipoprotein (a) decreases on treatment with hydrosoluble coenzyme Q10 in patients with coronary artery disease: discovery of a new role. *Int J Cardiol* 68 (1999): 23–29.

43. Singh, R.B., et al. Randomized double-blind placebo-controlled trial of coenzyme Q10 in patients with acute myocardial infarction. *Cardiovasc Drugs Ther* 12 (1998): 347–53.

44. Soja, A.M., and S.A. Mortensen. Treatment of chronic cardiac insufficiency with coenzyme Q10, results of meta-analysis in controlled clinical trials. *Ugeskr Laeger* 159 (1997): 7302–8; Gaby, A.R. The role of coenzyme Q10 in clinical medicine: part II. Cardiovascular disease, hypertension, diabetes mellitus and infertility. *Alt Med Rev* 1 (1996):1 68–75 [review]; Mortensen, S.A. Perspectives on therapy of cardiovascular diseases with coenzyme Q10 (ubiquinone). *Clin Invest* 71, suppl. (1993): s116–s123 [review].

45. Castano, G., et al. Effects of policosanol and pravastatin on lipid profile, platelet aggregation and endothelemia in older hypercholesterolemic patients. *Int J Clin Pharmacol Res* 19 (1999): 105–16; Mas, R., et al. Effects of policosanol in patients with type II hypercholesterolemia and additional coronary risk factors. *Clin Pharmacol Ther* 65 (1999): 439–47; Fernandez, J.C., et al. Comparison of the efficacy, safety and tolerability of policosanol versus fluvastatin in elderly hypercholesterolaemic women. *Clin Drug Invest* 21 (2001): 103–13.

46. Menendez, R., et al. Cholesterol-lowering effect of policosanol on rabbits with hypercholesterolaemia induced by a wheat starch-casein diet. *Br J Nutr* 77 (1997): 923–32.

47. Arruzazabala, M.L., et al. Comparative study of policosanol, aspirin and the combination therapy policosanol-aspirin on platelet aggregation in healthy volunteers. *Pharmacol Res* 36 (1997): 293–97.

48. Castano, G., et al. Effects of policosanol on postmenopausal women with type II hypercholesterolemia. *Gynecol Endocrinol* 14 (2000): 187–95; Mas, R., et al. Effects of policosanol in patients with type II hypercholesterolemia and additional coronary risk factors. *Clin Pharmacol Ther* 65 (1999): 439–47; Castano, G., et al. Effects of policosanol in hypertensive patients with type II hypercholesterolemia. *Curr Ther Res* 57 (1996): 691–99.

49. Silagy, C., A.W. Neil. A meta-analysis of the effect of garlic on blood pressure. *J Hypertension* 12 (1994): 463–68.

50. Silagy, C., and A. Neil. Garlic as a lipid-lowering agent—a meta-analysis. *J R Coll Physicians London* 28 (1994): 39–45; Warshafsky, S., R.S. Kamer, and S.L. Sivak. Effect of garlic on total serum cholesterol. A meta-analysis. *Ann Intern Med* 119 (1993): 599–605; Steiner, M., et al. A double-blind crossover study in moderately hypercholesterolemic men that compared the effect of aged garlic extract and placebo administration on blood lipids. *Am J Clin Nutr* 64 (1996): 866–70.

51. Holzgartner, J., U. Schmidt, U. Kuhn. Comparison of the efficacy of a garlic preparation vs. bezafibrate. *Arzneim-Forsch Drug Res* 421(992): 1473–77.

52. Kleijnen, J., P. Knipschild, and G. Ter Riet. Garlic, onion and cardiovascular risk factors: a review of the evidence from human experiments with emphasis on commercially available preparations. *Br J Clin Pharmacol* 28 (1989): 535–44.

53. Koscienlny, J., et al. The antiatherosclerotic effect of *Allium sativum. Atherosclerosis* 144 (1999): 237–49.

54. Agarwal, R.C., et al. Clinical trial of gugulipid new hypolipidemic agent of plant origin in primary hyperlipidemia. *Indian J Med Res* 84 (1986): 626–34.

55. Nityanand, S., J.S. Srivastava, and O.P. Asthana. Clinical trials with Gugulipid—a new hypolipidemic agent. *J Assoc Phys India* 37 (1989): 323–28.

56. Ripsin, C.M., et al. Oat products and lipid lowering: a meta-analysis. *JAMA* 267 (1992): 3317–25.

57. Holme, I. An analysis of randomized trials evaluating the effect of cholesterol reduction on total mortality and coronary heart disease incidence. *Circulation* 82 (1990): 1916–24.

Chapter 19 Diabetes: Stop the Epidemic

1. Canadian Diabetes Association. *The Prevalence and Cost of Diabetes.* Toronto: Canadian Diabetes Association, June 2000.

2. American Diabetes Association. "Basic Diabetes Information: Facts and Figures." <www.diabetes.org>. American Diabetes Association. 11 June 2002 <www.diabetes.org/main/application/commercewf?origin=*.jsp&event=link(B1)>.

3. American Diabetes Association. "Diabetes and Seniors." <www.diabetes.org>. American Diabetes Association. 12 June 2002 <www.diabetes.org/main/application/commercewf?origin=*.jsp&event=link(B4_4)>.

4. Centers for Disease Control. "Diabetes Rates Rise Another 6 Percent in 1999." <www.cdc.gov>. Centers for Disease Control, National Center for Chronic Disease Prevention and Health Promotion. 12 June 2002 <www.cdc.gov/nccdphp/dnpa/press/archive/diabetes_rates.htm>.

5. World Health Organization. "Fact Sheet No. 138, Diabetes Mellitus." <www.who.int>. World Health Organization. 12 June 2002 <www.who.int/inf-fs/en/fact138.html>.

6. American Diabetes Association. "Basic Diabetes Information: Diabetes and Seniors." <www.diabetes.org>. American Diabetes Association. 12 June 2002 <www.diabetes.org/main/application/commercewf?origin=*.jsp&event=link(B4_4)>.

7. American Diabetes Association. "Basic Diabetes Information: Diabetes in Children." <www.diabetes.org>. American Diabetes Association. 15 June 2002 <www.diabetes.org/main/application/commercewf?origin=*.jsp&event=link(B4_3)>.

8. Flier, J.S. "Obesity." In *Joslin's Diabetes Mellitus*, edited by R.C. Kahn and G.C. Weir. 13th ed. Philadelphia: Lea & Febiger, 1994. 351–61.

9. The Diabetes Control and Complications Trial Research Group. The effect of intensive treatment of diabetes on the development and progression of long-term complications in insulin-dependent diabetes mellitus. *N Engl J Med* 329 (1993): 977–86.

10. Pan, X.R., et al. Effects of diet and exercise in preventing NIDDM in people with impaired glucose tolerance: the Da Qing IGT and Diabetes Study. *Diabetes Care* 20 (1997): 537–44.

11. Salmeron, J., et al. Dietary fibre, glycemic load, and risk of non-insulin-dependent diabetes mellitus in women. *JAMA* 277 (1997): 472–77; Salmeron, J., et al. Dietary fibre, glycemic load, and risk of NIDDM in men. *Diabetes Care* 20 (1997): 545–50; Feskens, E.J., et al. Dietary factors determining diabetes and impaired glucose tolerance: a 20-year follow-up of the Finnish and Dutch cohorts of the Seven Countries Study. *Diabetes Care* 18 (1995): 1104–12.

12. American Diabetes Association. Evidence-based nutrition principles and recommendations for the treatment and prevention of diabetes and related complications. *Diabetes Care* 25, suppl. 1 (2002): S50–S60.

13. Madrick, B. Canadian Diabetes Association. "Carbohydrate Counting." Canadian Diabetes Association. 16 June 2002 <www.diabetes.ca/Section_About/carbcount.asp>.

14. Wolk, A., et al. Long-term intake of dietary fiber and decreased risk of coronary heart disease among women. *JAMA* 281 (1999): 1998–2004; Wood, P.J., et al. Comparisons of viscous properties of oat and guar gum and the effects of these and oat bran on glycemic index. *J Agric Food Chem* 38 (1990): 753–757.

15. Wood, P.J., et al. Effect of dose and modification of viscous properties of oat gum on plasma glucose and insulin following an oral glucose load. *B J Nutr* 72 (1994): 731–43.

16. Glore, S.R., et al. "Soluble fiber and serum lipids: a literature review." *Journal of the American Dieticians Association* 94 (1994): 425–36.

17. Wursch, P., and R.X. Pi-Sunyer. The role of viscous soluble fiber in the metabolic control of diabetes. *Diabetes Care* 20 (1997): 1774–80.

18. Liu, S., et al. Whole-grain consumption and risk of coronary artery disease: results from the Nurses' Health Study. *Am J Clin Nutr* 70 (1999): 412–19.

19. American Diabetes Association. Evidence-based nutrition principles. S50–S60.

20. Karter, A.J., et al. Insulin sensitivity and abdominal obesity in African-American, Hispanic, and non-Hispanic white men and women. *Diabetes* 45 (1996): 1547–55; Park, K.S., et al. Intra-abdominal fat is associated with decreased insulin sensitivity in healthy young men. *Metabolism* 40 (1991): 600–603.

21. Long, S.D., et al. Weight loss in severely obese subjects prevents the progression of impaired glucose tolerance to type II diabetes. *Diabetes Care* 17 (1994): 372; Pi-Sunyer, F.X. Weight and non-insulin-dependent diabetes mellitus. *Am J Clin Nutr* 63, suppl. (1996): 426S–29S.

22. Paolisso, G., et al. Pharmacologic doses of vitamin E improve insulin action in healthy subjects and non-insulin dependent diabetic patients. *Am J Clin Nutr* 57 (1993): 650–56.

23. Jain, S.K., et al. Effect of modest vitamin E supplementation on blood glycated hemoglobin and triglyceride levels and red cell indices in type I diabetic patients. *J Am Coll Nutr* 15 (1996): 458–61.

24. Ross, W.M., et al. Modelling cortical cataractogenesis: 3. In vivo effects of vitamin E on cataractogenesis in diabetic rats. *Canadian Journal of Ophthalmology* 17 (1982): 61; Bursell, S.E., et al. High-dose vitamin E supplementation normalizes retinal blood flow and creatinine clearance in patients with type I diabetes. *Diabetes Care* 22 (1999): 1245–51.

25. Eriksson, J., and A. Kohvakka. Magnesium and ascorbic acid supplementation in diabetes mellitus. *Ann Nutr Metab* 39 (1995): 217–23; Paolisso, G., et al. Metabolic benefits deriving from chronic vitamin C supplementation in aged non-insulin dependent diabetics. *J Am Coll Nutr* 14 (1995): 387–92.

26. Davie, S.J., B.J. Gould, and J.S. Yudkin. Effect of vitamin C on glycosylation of proteins. *Diabetes* 41 (1992): 167–73.

27. Will, J.C., and T. Tyers. Does diabetes mellitus increase the requirement for vitamin C? *Nutr Rev* 54 (1996): 193–202 [review].

28. Branch, D.R. High-dose vitamin C supplementation increases plasma glucose. *Diabetes Care* 22 (1999): 1218 [letter].

29. McCann, V.J., and R.E. Davis, Serum pyridoxal concentrations in patients with diabetic neuropathy. *Australia and New Zealand Journal of Medicine* 8 (1978): 259–61.

30. Yamane, K., et al. Clinical efficacy of intravenous plus oral mecobalamin in patients with peripheral neuropathy using vibration perception thresholds as an indicator of improvement. *Current Therapeutic Research* 56 (1995): 656–70 [review]; Kuwabara, S., et al. Intravenous methylcobalamin treatment for uremic and diabetic neuropathy in chronic hemodialysis patients. *Intern Med J* 38 (1999): 472–75.

31. Koutsikos, D., B. Agroyannis, and H. Tzanatos-Exarchou. Biotin for diabetic peripheral neuropathy. *Biomed Pharmacother* 44 (1990): 511–14.

32. Maebashi, M., et al. Therapeutic evaluation of the effect of biotin on hyperglycemia in patients with non-insulin dependent diabetes mellitus. *Journal of Clinical Biochemical Nutrition* 14 (1993): 211–18.

33. Gaby, A.R., and J.V. Wright. "Diabetes." In *Nutritional Therapy in Medical Practice: Reference Manual and Study Guide*. Kent, WA, 1996. 54–64 [review].

34. Lee, N.A., and C.A. Reasner. Beneficial effect of chromium supplementation on serum triglyceride levels in NIDDM. *Diabetes Care* 17 (1994): 1449–52; Hermann, J., et al. Effects of chromium or copper supplementation on plasma lipids, plasma glucose and serum insulin in adults over age fifty. *Journal of Nutrition for the Elderly* 18 (1998): 27–45.

35. Paolisso, G., et al. Magnesium and glucose homeostasis. *Diabetologia* 33 (1990): 511–14 [review].

36. Eibl, N.L., et al. Hypomagnesemia in type II diabetes: effect of a 3-month replacement therapy. *Diabetes Care* 18 (1995): 188.

37. Konrad, T., et al. Alpha lipoic acid treatment decreases serum lactate and pyruvate concentrations and improves glucose effectiveness in lean and obese patients with type 2 diabetes. *Diabetes Care* 22 (1999): 280–87.

38. Reljanovic, M., et al. Treatment of diabetic polyneuropathy with the antioxidant thioctic acid (alpha-lipoic acid): a two year multicenter randomized double-blind placebo-controlled trial (ALADIN II). Alpha Lipoic Acid in Diabetic Neuropathy. *Free Radic Res* 31 (1999): 171–79.

39. Scharrer, A., and M. Ober. Anthocyanoside in der Behandlung von Retinopathien. *Klin Monatsblatt Augenheilk* 178 (1981): 386–89.

40. Shanmugasundaram, E.R.B., et al. Use of *Gymnema sylvestre* leaf extract in the control of blood glucose insulin-dependent diabetes mellitus. *J Ethnopharmacol* 30 (1990): 281–94.

41. Baskaran, K., et al. Antidiabetic effect of a leaf extract from *Gymnema sylvestre* in non-insulin-dependent diabetes mellitus patients. *J Ethnopharmacol* 30 (1990): 295–305.

42. Zhang, T., et al. Ginseng root: Evidence for numerous regulatory peptides and insulinotropic activity. *Biomedical Research* 11 (1990): 49–54; Suzuki, Y., and H. Hikino. Mechanisms of hypoglycemic activity of panaxans A and B, glycans of *Panax ginseng* roots: effects on plasma levels, secretion, sensitivity and binding of insulin in mice. *Phytother Res* 3 (1989): 20–24.

43. Sotaniemi, E.A., E. Haapakoski, and A. Rautio. Ginseng therapy in non-insulin-dependent diabetic patients. *Diabetes Care* 18 (1995): 1373–75.

Chapter 20 Cancer: Genetically Programmed or Environmentally Acquired?

1. *Cancer Facts & Figures 2002.* Special section, "Colorectal Cancer and Early Detection." Atlanta, GA: American Cancer Society, 2002.

2. National Cancer Institute of Canada. *Canadian Cancer Statistics 2002.* Toronto, April 2002.

3. *Cancer Facts & Figures 2002*; National Cancer Institute of Canada.

4. Lichtenstein, P., et al. Environmental and heritable factors in the causation of cancer: analyses of cohorts of twins from Sweden, Denmark and Finland. *N Engl J Med* 343 (2000): 78–85.

5. *Cancer Facts & Figures 2001.* Special section, "Obesity." Atlanta, GA: American Cancer Society, 2001.

6. Thune, I., et al. Physical activity and the risk of breast cancer. *N Engl J Med* 336 (1 May 1997): 1269–75.

7. Thomas, C.B. Precursors of premature disease and death: the predictive potential of habits and family attitudes. *Ann Intern Med* 85 (1976): 653–58.

8. Barefoot, J.C., et al. Hostility, coronary heart disease incidence, and total mortality: 25-year follow-up study of 255 physicians. *Psychosom Med* 45.1 (1983): 59–63.

9. Schleifer, S.J., et al. Suppression of lymphocyte stimulation following bereavement. *JAMA* 250.3 (1983): 374 –77.

10. Bartrop, R.W., et al. Depressed lymphocyte function after bereavement. *Lancet* 1977 1:8016 pages 843 to 836

11. Kiecolt-Glaser, J.K. et al. Psychological modifiers of immunocompetence in medical students. *Psychosom Med* 46.1 (1984): 7–14.

12. Reynolds, P., and G.A. Kaplan. "Social Connections and Cancer: A Prospective Study of Alameda County Residents." Paper presented at the annual meeting of the Society of Behavioral Medicine, San Francisco, CA, March 1996; Berkman, L., and S. Syme. Social networks, host resistance, and mortality: a nine-year follow-up study of Alameda County residents. *Am J Epidemiol* 109 (1982): 186–204.

13. World Cancer Research and American Institute for Cancer Research Report: *Food, Nutrition and the Prevention of Cancer: A Global Perspective.* Washington, DC: American Institute for Cancer Research, 1997. 506–7.

14. Ames, B.N. Micronutrients prevent cancer and delay aging. *Toxicol Lett* 102.3 (18 Dec. 1998): 5–18 [review].

15. G.F. Combs, Jr., "Quantifying Vitamin Needs." In *The Vitamins: Fundamental Aspects in Nutrition and Health,* 2nd ed. San Diego, CA: Academic Press, 1998, 512–34.

16. Shamberger, R.J., and D.V. Frost. Possible preventative effect of selenium on human cancer. *Can Med Assoc J* 100 (1969): 682–86; Shamberger, R.J. Relationship of selenium to cancer: inhibitory effect of selenium on carcinogenesis. *J Natl Cancer Inst* 44.4 (April 1970): 931–36; Combs, G.F., Jr. Impact of selenium and cancer-prevention findings on the nutrition-health paradigm. *Nutr Cancer* 40.1 (2001): 6–11; Combs, G.F., Jr., L.C. Clark, and B.W. Turnbull. An analysis of cancer prevention by selenium. *Biofactors* 14.1–4 (2001): 153–9 [review]; Clark, L.C., et al. Effects of selenium supplementation for cancer prevention in patients with carcinoma of the skin: a randomized controlled trial. *JAMA* 276.24 (1996): 1957–63; Blot, W.J., et al., The Linxian trials: mortality rates by vitamin-mineral group. *Am J Clin Nutr* 62 (1995): S1424–S1426.

17. Block, G., B. Patterson, and A. Subar. Fruit, vegetables, and cancer prevention: a review of the epidemiological evidence. *Nutr Cancer* 18 (1992): 1–29; Steinmetz, K.A., and J.D. Patter. Vegetables, fruit, and cancer prevention. *J Am Diet Assoc* 96 (1996): 1027–39 [review]; Willet, W.C., and D. Trichopoulos. Nutrition and cancer: a summary of the evidence. *Cancer Causes Control* 7 (1996): 178–80.

18. Willet, W.C. "Diet, Nutrition, and the Prevention of Cancer." In *Modern Nutrition in Health and Disease,* edited by M.E. Shils et al. 9th ed. Baltimore, MD: Lippincott Williams & Wilkins, 1999. 1243–53.

19. Simone, C.B., N.L. Simone, and C.B. Simone, Jr. Fibre consumption reduces the risk of colorectal cancer. *International Journal of Integrative Medicine* 2.4 (July/August 2000): 38–43.

20. Simpopoulos, A.P. The Mediterranean diets: what is so special about the diet of Greece? The scientific evidence. *J Nutr* 131, suppl. 11 (Nov. 2001): 3065S–73S [review].

21. Chatenoud, L., et al. Refined-cereal intake and risk of selected cancers in Italy. *Am J Clin Nutr* 70.6 (Dec. 1999): 1107–10.

22. Norton, H.A., and R.R. Butrum. Maintaining an energy balance lowers cancer risk: new review finds unexpected effect of excess insulin. *American Institute for Cancer Research Science News,* no. 23 (Mar. 2002).

23. Gdanski, R. *Cancer: Cause, Cure and Cover-up.* Grimsby, ON: Nadex Publishing, 2000.

24. Zheng, W., et al. Well-done meat intake and the risk of breast cancer. *J Natl Cancer Inst* 90.22 (1998): 1724–29.

25. Nerurkar, P.V., et al. Effects of marinating with Asian marinades or western barbecue sauce on PhIP and MelQx formation in barbecued beef. *Nutr Cancer* 34 (1999): 147–52; Salmon, C.P., et al. Effects of marinating on heterocyclic amine carcinogen formation in grilled chicken. *Food Chem Toxicol* 35 (1997): 433–41.

26. Mitchell, T. Prostate cancer and I3C. *Life Extension* May 2002.

27. National Toxicology Program, and the National Institute of Environmental Health Services under the National Institutes of Health. *The 9th Report on Carcinogens 2000. Rev. ed.* Bethesda, MD., 2001.

28. Hulley, S., et al. Randomized trial of estrogen plus progestin for secondary prevention of coronary heart disease in postmenopausal women. *JAMA* 280 (1998): 605–13; D'Agostino, R.B., Jr. Debate: the slippery slope of surrogate outcomes. *Curr Control Trials Cardiovasc Med* 1 (2000): 76–78;

Simon, J.A., et al. Postmenopausal hormone therapy and risk of stroke: the Heart and Estrogen-progestin Replacement Study (HERS). *Circulation* 103.5 (6 Feb. 2001): 638–42; Contreras, I., and D. Parra. Estrogen replacement therapy and the prevention of coronary heart disease in post-menopausal women. *Am J Health Syst Pharm* 57.21 (1 Nov. 2000): 1963–68, quiz 1969–71 [review]; Colditz, G.A., et al. The use of estrogens and the risk of breast cancer in postmenopausal women. *NEJM* 332.24 (15 June 1995): 1589–93.

29. Torisu, M., et al. Significant prolongation of disease-free period gained by oral polysaccharide K (PSK) administration after curative surgical operation of colorectal cancer. *Cancer Immunol Immunother* 31 (1990): 261–68; Nakazato, H., et al. Efficacy of immunochemotherapy as adjuvant treatment after curative resection of gastric cancer. *Lancet* 343 (1994): 1122–26; Hayakawa, K., et al. Effect of krestin (PSK) as adjuvant treatment on the prognosis after radical radiotherapy in patients with non-small cell lung cancer. *Anticancer Res* 13 (1993): 1815–20; Iino, Y., et al. Immunochemotherapies versus chemotherapy as adjuvant treatment after curative resection of operable breast cancer. *Anticancer Res* 15 (1995): 2907–12.

30. Colodny, L., et al. Results of a study to evaluate the use of propax to reduce adverse effects of chemotherapy. *JANA* 3.2 (Summer 2000): 17–25; Block, J.B., and S. Evans. Clinical evidence supporting cancer risk reduction with antioxidants and implications for diet and supplementation. *JANA* 3.3. (Fall 2000): 6–16; Blaylock, R.L. A review of conventional cancer prevention and treatment and the adjunctive use of nutraceutical supplements and antioxidants: is there a danger or a significant benefit? *JANA* 3.3 (Fall 2000): 17–35; Block, J.B., and S. Evans. A review of recent results addressing the potential interactions of antioxidants with cancer drug therapy. *JANA* 4.1 (Spring 2001): 11–20; Lamson, D.W., and M.S. Brignall. Antioxidants in cancer therapy: their actions and interactions with oncologic therapies. *Altern Med Rev* 4 (1999): 304–29; Lamson, D.W., and M.S. Brignall. Antioxidants and cancer therapy II: quick reference guide. *Altern Med Rev* 5 (2000): 152–63.

INDEX

peptic ulcers, 79, 80
perimenopause, 124
Phase 2™, 108
phosphatidylcholine, 151
phosphatidylserine, 151
phosphorus, 115
physical activity. *See* exercise
phytochemicals, benefits of, 186
pituitary gland, 10
plant sterols and sterolins, 99
policosanol, 160–161
pollen extract, 141
polyphenols, 142
poor diets
    caffeine, 21
    overeating, 21–22
    refined grains, 19
    sugar consumption, 19–20
    trans fatty acids, 20
positive attitude, 35–36
prayer, 39
pregnenolone, 59
presbycusis, 121
probiotics, 98
the prostate
    benign prostatic hyperplasia. *See* benign
      prostatic hyperplasia (BPH)
    function, 134
    maintaining prostate health, 139–140
    prostate-specific antigen (PSA) test, 136
    prostatitis, 134–135, 142–143
prostatitis, 134–135, 142–143
protein, 48–49, 168
psychological factors for successful aging, 26–28
psyllium, 169
Pygeum africanum extract, 141
pyridoxine, 66

Q
quality of foods, 52
quantity of food, 53–54
quercetin, 89

R
Rate of Living Theory of Aging, 7–8
rating of perceived exertion (RPE) scale, 43
ReCleanse, 77–78
red clover extract, 131
refined grains, 19, 176
relaxation response, 38
resistance training, 44–46, 105–106
rosemary, 80
Rubner, Max, 7

S
S-adenosyl-L-methionine, 151
saboteurs of health. *See* health threats
saturated fats, 51, 168
saw palmetto, 140
Schambaugh, George, 24–25
Sears, Barry, 103
secondhand smoke, 16
sedentary lifestyle, 23
selective estrogen receptor modulators (SERMs),
  116
selenium, 67, 159–160, 175
self-esteem, 27
Selye, Hans, 17, 35
sex hormone-binding globulin (SHBG), 137
sexual performance, 143
sexuality, and menopause, 125
silicon, 115
simple carbohydrates, 49
sleep
    and depression, 19
    lack of, 18–19
    statistics, 19
    and stress, 38
slippery elm bark, 80
smoking
    adverse effects of nicotine, 16
    cadmium, 138
    and cardiovascular disease, 154–155
    mortality statistics, 15
    quitting, and longevity, 16
    secondhand effects, 16
Snowdon, David, 35
soy foods, 104, 113, 141
soybeans, 53, 132
Spears, Tom, 29
spirituality
    and stress, 39
    and successful aging, 26–27
St. John's wort, 131, 151–152
staphylococcus, 99
statistics. *See* health statistics
sterols and sterolins. *See* plant sterols and
  sterolins
stevia, 20
stiffening of the brain, 146
stinging nettle, 90, 140–141
stress
    adaptogens and, 63–64
    aging brain and, 145–146
    and aging process, 35
    and beneficial bacteria in colon, 73
    and benign prostatic hyperplasia (BPH), 137
    and cancer, 174–175